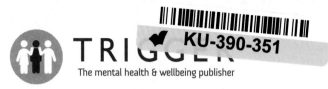

The mental health & wellbeing publisher

www.triggerpublishing.com

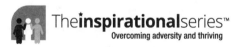

The**inspirational**series™
Overcoming adversity and thriving

Barber Talk
Taking Pride in Men's Mental Health

BY TOM CHAPMAN

We are proud to introduce The**inspirational**series™. Part of the Trigger family of innovative mental health books, The**inspirational**series™ tells the stories of the people who have battled and beaten mental health issues. For more information visit: www.triggerpublishing.com

THE AUTHOR

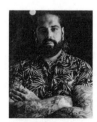

Tom Chapman is an award-winning barber, author, public speaker, global ambassador and international educator. He has educated and performed all over the UK, Europe, USA, Canada, Asia and Brazil. A multi-published session stylist and platform artist, Tom has even had his work grace the front cover of industry magazines, including *HJ Men*.

Believing that the barbershop is a great, safe place for men to talk, Tom founded The Lions Barber Collective in September 2015. The Lions are an international group of barbers raising awareness for suicide prevention. Tom has delivered a TEDx talk on the subject and has been featured on multiple national and international media outlets, including the BBC. In 2017 Tom received a Points of Light award from the UK Prime minister for his outstanding volunteer work, and he looks forward to meeting Prince William in 2019.

Tom published his first book, *The Barber Boom*, in 2018.

First published in Great Britain 2019 by Trigger

Trigger is a trading style of Shaw Callaghan Ltd & Shaw Callaghan 23 USA, INC.

The Foundation Centre

Navigation House, 48 Millgate, Newark

Nottinghamshire NG24 4TS UK

www.triggerpublishing.com

Copyright © Tom Chapman 2019

British Library Cataloguing in Publication Data

A CIP catalogue record for this book is available upon request
from the British Library

ISBN: 978-1-912478-21-7

This book is also available in the following e-Book and Audio formats:

MOBI: 978-1-912478-24-8
EPUB: 978-1-912478-22-4
PDF: 978-1-912478-23-1

Tom Chapman has asserted his right under the Copyright,
Design and Patents Act 1988 to be identified as the author of this work

Cover design and typeset by Fusion Graphic Design Ltd

Printed and bound in Great Britain by Clays Ltd, Elcograf S.p.A

Paper from responsible sources

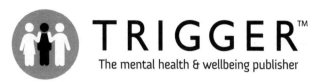

TRIGGER™

The mental health & wellbeing publisher

www.triggerpublishing.com

Thank you for purchasing this book.
You are making an incredible difference.

Proceeds from all Trigger books go directly to
The Shaw Mind Foundation, a global charity that focuses
entirely on mental health. To find out more about
The Shaw Mind Foundation visit,
www.shawmindfoundation.org

MISSION STATEMENT

Our goal is to make help and support available for every
single person in society, from all walks of life.
We will never stop offering hope. These are our promises.

Trigger and The Shaw Mind Foundation

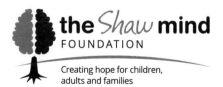

the *Shaw* **mind**
FOUNDATION

Creating hope for children,
adults and families

A NOTE FROM THE SERIES EDITOR

The Inspirational range from Trigger brings you genuine stories about our authors' experiences with mental health problems.

Some of the stories in our Inspirational range will move you to tears. Some will make you laugh. Some will make you feel angry, or surprised, or uplifted. Hopefully they will all change the way you see mental health problems.

These are stories we can all relate to and engage with. Stories of people experiencing mental health difficulties and finding their own ways to overcome them with dignity, humour, perseverance and spirit.

Tom's work in the community is commendable, as is his drive to break through the stigma surrounding mental health problems, and his Lions Barber Collective strives to emulate this around the world. However, Tom's story is of how this all started, and it began with the loss of a friend to suicide, for which he was completely unprepared.

His story tells the tale of how, through his work as a barber, Tom realised the need for men to be able to talk to one another about how they were feeling; he himself had had no idea that his friend had been feeling so low. This drove him to talk to his clients whilst they were in the chair, and to encourage other barbers to do the same in the hopes that they could help reduce the high suicide rate among men. Barber Talk is a shining example of how we can all open up conversation around mental illness.

This is our Inspirational range. These are our stories. We hope you enjoy them. And most of all, we hope that they will educate and inspire you. That's what this range is all about.

Lauren Callaghan,
Co-founder and Lead Consultant Psychologist at Trigger

This book is for my family, for always standing by and supporting me. For my phenomenal wife, Tenneille, for driving me forward and enabling me to be more than I ever thought I could be. And finally, for my two boys – I hope that by the time they are young men the stigma and taboo around men's mental health is long gone, and they are free to be whoever they want to be.

Disclaimer: Some names and identifying details have been changed to protect the privacy of individuals.

Trigger Warning: This book contains references to suicide and suicidal thoughts.

INTRODUCTION

Ever since I can remember – at least since I started working in the hair industry as a fresh-faced 18-year-old – there has been a saying bandied about: 'We aren't just hairdressers; we're psychologists and counsellors too.' Sometimes a hairdresser is referred to as "a poor man's psychologist".

It's always said as a joke, but hairdressers are well aware that female clients sometimes find it helpful to offload to them while sitting in the chair.

But is this the same for men?

As a unisex stylist, I can say from my experience at least that this notion *has* moved across into the barber world, and that men certainly tell all in that chair too. Having been behind the chair for the last 15 years, I have heard many, many stories – some good, some bad, and a lot of them powerful. There have been love triangles, affairs, marriage proposal plans, births, miscarriages, anniversaries, redundancies, promotions, surprise celebrations, funerals, breakdowns, breakthroughs, lottery winners, bankruptcy, coming out, losses, depression, adventure, diagnosis of cancer, beating cancer, new love, admiration – and there are more that I've not mentioned! There are some clients whose entire lives I have been privy to – men who were single when I met them, who then told me about their first date, their planned proposal, their stag-do escapades, pregnancy announcements, the births of their children, and their ongoing adventure through life. I feel honoured that they want to share all this with me, I really am lucky and privileged to have such a wonderful career and position.

Now, I'm not saying that everyone will open up like this, and that is perfectly fine. But some do. And that is why it is so important that we give as many people as many opportunities to open up in as many different places as possible. For some this feels right, and I know for a fact that it can make a difference and save a life.

I have been incredibly public about the fact that it is okay to talk to me, and that I will listen without judgement and with empathy. In my opinion, this is the single biggest thing I have done. It is because I did this that lives were saved.

You have a friend in me.

CHAPTER 1

PAUSE FOR THOUGHT

In February of 2017, after I did a piece for BBC Radio, I was asked if I would be interested in taking part in a programme called *Pause for Thought*. I'm not going to lie, I was flattered to be asked, but I was unaware of what *Pause for Thought* was. Luckily the gentleman from the BBC explained what it was – an early-morning radio segment lasting two or three minutes. I did a little bit of research into previous speakers so that I would have an idea of what they were expecting, and to be honest I was a bit shocked. All their guests were well-respected and intelligent people. *Why the hell would he ask me?* I thought. *God only knows why!*

But he had asked me, and it was such an honour. I like to say yes to most things, as I never know what further opportunities can come from them (even though I am often terrified after I have committed to something!). And so having agreed, I went home and told my family. My parents were really impressed and my wife, like me, needed an explanation of what it actually was. But all of the older generation in my family were incredibly proud, and that is always lovely for me.

This meant that I now had to come up with a separate story for each morning, one that would encourage those listening to

Pause for Thought. It wasn't an easy task but I decided to draw from personal experience and knowledge.

It all started on a Monday morning with a trip to the local BBC Studios in Plymouth, where I was invited to record one week's worth of *Pause for Thought*. The building is in a residential area, an old grand house which has been built upon and added to over the years. It was early doors because the first piece I would record would be live that day and it was to go out just after six o'clock in the morning. Because of this it was dark and there weren't many people around. I walked nervously up to the big front doors and pressed the buzzer to get in before heading up to a small waiting area outside the studio. It was totally surreal to hear all the DJs working and listening to the jingles going on – watching the workings of BBC Radio wasn't something I expected to do in my lifetime!

I was a little nervous about being on live radio. Would my stories be good enough, especially compared to the standard of those who had come before me? The DJ made me feel at ease though, and after a little chit-chat we went straight into the first story. It just rolled off my tongue pretty easily – what a relief it was when it was over! I did need to record the other six stories for the rest of the week, but thankfully not live. I ended up messing the last couple of stories up a little, but luckily we were able to just go back and record them again.

Once I was done, I felt a huge sense of relief and achievement. These six stories were played out every morning one week in 2017, and now here they are as their own chapters, scattered throughout this book.

I hope they all can help you pause for thought.

CHAPTER 2

FEELING SAFE

I was born the first of three children in Maidstone, Kent in 1984, where I spent the first 10 years of my life. I come from what I would consider a fairly stable family unit, with parents who were brilliant role models.

Apparently, I was a very easy child. I was calm, I wasn't a fussy eater, I slept, and was more than happy to sit and cuddle for long periods of time. From what I can gather, I was pretty content as a kid.

My brother Joe – who arrived a year after I was born – was completely different. He was a bad sleeper for one, and he had a lot more energy than me. I think I lulled my parents into a false sense of security. How many times have we heard that story? 'Our first was so easy, so we decided we should definitely have another child ...'

Joe is truly brilliant. He didn't speak until he was around five years old, and the doctors thought that there was a chance he might never talk. But then he had a moment while watching 80's children's TV show, *Rainbow*. He mimicked a clock "tick-tocking" and that was it – he never looked back! He attended speech therapy and got a lot of help for it. (In fact, interestingly we are now experiencing a similar trait in my eldest son, who is saying *some* words, but would rather communicate onomatopoeically. I have been assured that he will be fine and there is nothing to worry about though.)

Growing up, my brother and I spent a lot of time together playing football. During the school holidays we'd play from eight in the morning until eight at night in our full Arsenal kits, and as Arsenal supporters we had some fun imitating Thierry Henry, Dennis Bergkamp, and Patrick Vieira, our favourite players. When we couldn't go out to play football, we would spend our time playing FIFA games on the PlayStation, often with friends. This was back when you all had to be in the same room if you wanted to play each other. (This sudden thought about technology comes because I am currently sitting on a plane, flying over the Atlantic while using Wi-Fi. How crazy is that? The future is here!)

And when we weren't playing football of some kind, we would be fishing, swimming in the sea, jumping from the pier, running in the glens, playing up the mountain, or making dens.

As we grew up into our teens and early twenties, we spent a lot of time together out and about on the scene, hanging out at festivals and parties of all shapes and sizes. We had friendship groups that overlapped, and although we were personally into the alternative scene, our groups were pretty diverse in terms of tastes and opinions, and that made for a lot of fun.

I believe that the diversity, acceptance, and openness within the small alternative scene definitely left us all with open minds. Devon is a small place and the area of Torbay even smaller; factor that in with the reality that most people our age had gone away to university, and it was a pretty tight-knit group of misfits, really. There were punk rockers, metalheads, goths, and hippies, all with strong and differing opinions.

Many of our stories together are fun and interesting, and many of them involve some kind of danger – you know the ones. Some stories should never be retold, especially in a place where your parents can read them. (I know that mine will ask me now.) You know when you look back and think, *Jesus, what was I thinking? No one knew where I was, who I was with, or what I was doing. How am I still alive and not in some shallow grave somewhere?*

My little sister joined the family five years after I did, and that's where my parents stopped. Lucy will tell you it's because they reached perfection at that point, but my brother and I would beg to differ. When she was born, all I wanted to do was look after her. That's a complete 180-degree change in attitude compared to how I felt when my brother was born. I'm told my parents found me trying to hit Joe over the head with a saucepan when they first brought him home, and yet there are a lot of photos of me and Lucy as a baby in dens and in bed together.

Unfortunately, as we grew up, the five-year age gap started to seem pretty huge. It's really significant when you're a twelve-year-old boy and your sister is a seven-year-old girl. So, although we were an incredibly close family who spent a lot of time together, I spent a lot more time with my brother.

As we got older – especially around the ages of 22 and 17 – that began to change. My sister and I ended up spending a lot more time together, as friends as well as siblings. We'd moved to Devon at this point and we saw each other out and about at parties and down at the beach. When you live in a rural area, everyone seems to know everyone else and hang out together. Plus, when you're in your twenties and you have a sister who's five years younger than you, it results in a lot of girls coming around to your house all the time. My friends would always ask if we could invite them over.

One of my favourite things my friends and I did (and we did it a lot) was sit around a campfire, whether on a beach or in a woods somewhere, with some kind of cheap booze – usually cider – in one hand and a roll-up cigarette in the other. Here my sister and I would just talk to one another for hours. Those were really happy times. There was no need for anything else – nothing flashy, no big budgets, labels, or brands. We just had nature, fire, friends, and time talking and sharing with each other. Our conversations weren't always all meaningful or philosophical; in fact, I'm sure most of it was bullshit, but we really got to know each other this way.

Joe is now fluent in French and lives in Paris, where he's a lecturer in English. He's an inspiration to me – he knew what he wanted to do and went out there and got it, putting himself through an Open University course and moving to Paris by himself, throwing himself into the mix to ensure that he learnt French far more quickly. If that isn't brave, I don't know what is.

Nowadays, my sister is the family organiser. She keeps both my brother and me in the loop, and makes sure we stay updated whenever it comes to anything involving our family. I can see her being the head of the family one day. She is very dedicated and driven, which has made her the perfect child to go into business with our parents in their restaurants and fashion shops. She even puts them right from time to time!

Since as far back as I can remember, my parents have been entrepreneurs. Soon after I was born, my dad realised that he hated leaving me and my mum to go to work, so much so that they decided they needed to be their own bosses in order to have more flexibility and freedom. This led them to open a sandwich bar called Apple Food Company.

Nowadays there's a Subway on every corner, but in Maidstone in the mid-80s, a sandwich bar was pretty unusual for the time. And it was a huge success – until the recession hit in the early 90s.

My parents had to sell their home, their business, and an old school house in the south of France that they'd bought as a project to renovate (living in France had been their dream). This brought a lot of stress upon the family and, although I was young, I can remember it being incredibly hard for both my parents.

There's one memory from this time that really stands out in my mind. This vivid scene takes place at the foot of a large, freshly made white bed in the bedroom of a rented cottage. It was far smaller than the beautiful family home my parents had worked so hard for.

I was just 10 years old. I don't know all the ins and outs of what was going on between my parents at the time; I was just too young. I do, however, remember feeling scared that soon they would no longer be together. It gave me a deep sense of foreboding. I was worried about what would happen between my parents and what the future held for us financially. I couldn't remember ever having felt that way before. At that age it's hard to really understand those kinds of things. I mean, we had no idea about business or money and the stress it can cause. We had no idea at all. Why would we? Our parents had always protected us from all that. I can't even remember my parents ever arguing – we had always lived in a loving environment.

At that moment, in that cottage, my parents decided they would stay together. We would all relocate and find a new life, just us five, as a family unit. We all hugged and cried together, and in that moment I knew I was safe and that everything would be alright.

There are few feelings in life that are better than feeling safe. It's so important to us all, yet often taken for granted. That feeling has never gone away for me, and I value that safety every day. Just knowing that my parents are there for me is enough. Watching their strength, honesty, and openness – and seeing them be so loving with each other – helped me to develop my positive attitude towards emotions. I was always able to share with them how I felt. Our family has support and unconditional love, and it's is a luxury that many don't have.

And so we packed up our stuff and relocated to the Isle of Man. We had actually been to Cornwall as well just to check it out as a potential location, but for whatever reason we ended up on the little island in the middle of the Irish Sea. You probably couldn't find anywhere more different from the busy, highly populated, culturally diverse town of Maidstone. I moved from a huge school – one that had just sold part of its field to help widen the road in preparation for the development of the Channel Tunnel – to the tiny village school of Laxey, which had fewer than 100 students in the whole school.

My siblings and I had an utter ball! We were used to riding our bikes up and down a stretch of road between our house and our friend's house (about six doors up) with both mothers watching us all the time. But now we had complete freedom! My parents took on a huge restaurant in an old mill, and we lived in a flat above it. Across the road was a glen, which turned into a pine forest if you went deep enough into the canopy-covered paradise. Down the hill was a beach – in Kent we would have had to drive for hours on a Saturday in order to visit the beach – and directly behind the restaurant was an old-style electric tram station that took you to a never-ending supply of new glens, beaches, and even a mountain to explore.

To top it all off, once a year the island's population doubled, with bikers from all over the world travelling over for the TT Races, a motorbike road race with a huge history. This was always a sight to be seen. I can remember walking the promenade, deciding which bike I wanted to buy when I grew up.

(It was a Honda CBR with the street tiger custom paint. I still don't own a bike.)

I spent many, many hours of my childhood fishing, swimming, climbing, exploring, playing football, and making tree houses. Once, we even spent the entire school holidays venturing into and around the old mines at the base of the famous Laxey Wheel, searching for an alien that my brother, our friends and I insisted we'd spotted in the darkness. To say we were imaginative may be an understatement; I had a fantastic, old-school childhood, one that kept me innocent of the world's hardships. For that, I consider myself very lucky indeed.

I had a particularly strong bond with my Grandad Billy. I was the first grandchild in the family and I was a boy. Being a man's man with two daughters himself, he was incredibly happy about it. He was really into sports and he was handy too, making all sorts of things in his garage. I would help him garden and "mend" things, and I was always getting told off for climbing in the trees and jumping over his flower beds.

I have fond memories of his 1984 red Ford Escort Estate car – and admittedly I've even looked online to try to buy my own. I would love that. I can even remember the smell of it; it was similar to the smell of his garage workshop, probably because most of the stuff in his garage workshop got there via his car. The car itself was always parked on the road outside the house next to a garden wall made of brick. Grandad Billy would paint it with whatever colour paint he could get hold of for free, usually leftovers from some other project. He used some very interesting colours in his time. 'A blind man would love to see it,' he'd say if anyone ever questioned his colour choice. He had a good point.

Billy would always watch the cricket, or any other sport if cricket wasn't on that day. He would sit with his newspapers spread out across the whole surface of the kitchen table, eating "Grandad Billy biscuits" (custard creams – he'd always have some with his cup of tea).

He was also a key figure of the community, working at the local college and becoming heavily involved with the council. He organised so many events and was on the board for all sorts of things. He had connections in lots of areas and could get you anything you wanted. Not only was he head of the family and a phenomenal person, he was like a hero to me when I was little, always supporting our family in any way we needed.

Alongside the restaurant, my parents also had a film transport company. Dad was a location manager, and everything seemed to be going well for them. I really enjoyed my dad's time in the film industry; I spent a lot of hours on film sets, watching how movies were made and mingling with the likes of Catherine Zeta Jones and Mickey Rourke, although at the time I had no idea who these people really were. I think it was a time before celebrity culture had really kicked off, and it was way before social media and the age of the selfie. I was just living a dream, seeing how films were made and getting to stay up all night for night shoots, sitting in the back of pickup trucks and riding shotgun in big American campers. I even got to be an extra in a few films, which was really exciting. We even got paid for the pleasure!

I have memories of sitting in the small make-up and hair trailer in the middle of a field. Surrounding the trailer were all the other transport vehicles, from canteen buses to quad bikes. The trailer had those mirrors with the lights around them, like the ones you see on TV. I used to sit there and have my hair done in the same chair that film stars would sit in. That was pretty cool then, but it's even cooler looking back on it now. I don't suppose many people have had that opportunity.

Certain movies stood out for me. I loved watching the styling for films set in the war. There was even a film about George Best's life, in which they wore some pretty horrendous 1970's gear. One of my favourite memories is when they blew up a shed for a war movie called *The Brylcream Boys* which was about the Air Force in the Second World War. It was great fun. The sets they built were amazing! They had recreated a war camp up on an old air field in the north of the Isle of Man, with barbed-wire fences and huts and all the other fine details you'd expect for a movie. Dad had let me and Joe know in advance that this was going to happen, and so we had made the journey up with him to be on set. There was a lot of organising, and I can remember thinking that there was a hell of a lot of people there just to blow up a shed.

We were made to stand behind a clearance line, and obviously there could only be one take for this explosion, so even at that age I felt the tension and excitement in the air. Waiting for it to go up was kind of like when you're watching a scary movie and you're waiting for the jump scare, not knowing quite when it's going to happen. And of course there was silence, because they were filming. Then all of a sudden, *Boom!* There was a huge explosion and a ball of flames and black smoke.

I felt a big rush of excitement and adrenaline. In the air there was the smell of the smoke and whatever fuel they'd ignited.

When it was all over, I found the door knob – all black and charred from the explosion – not far from where I was standing. That door knob came home with me and sat by my bed for some time, serving as a reminder of the day and some of the great times I spent with my dad at work. It was so cool to go to work with my dad. Most of my mates had never seen where their dad worked, nor did they get to blow stuff up as part of their job!

Once I was asked to be an extra for a scene at a racetrack. As I was quite tall, they thought I could pass off as an adult, so they needed me to hold a beer and a cigarette. Or possibly they had a limited number of extras for the day and wanted to double me up as a child in one scene then a beer-swilling adult at the races in the next. Either way, I didn't care. I was more than happy to oblige! I got to hold the beer and even drink some of it, but my mum drew the line at that. I was probably about 13 at the time, and I felt pretty cool with a beer in hand.

I remember being on the set for an alien horror movie very well. I spent time with the 7ft actor inside the alien costume, and he happened to be an Arsenal fan. He towered over me while they showed us the animatronic puppet and fake saliva. They also blew up a foam alien on this movie – and I got to keep the foot in our attic "clubhouse" for years until it went mouldy with the damp.

Reading all of this back to myself, I find it strange that both my favourite films (that my parents worked on) are ones in which they blew stuff up. Is that a young boy thing? Maybe, although we humans *do* tend to like watching others destroy things ...

CHAPTER 3

IT'S ALL ABOUT CONFIDENCE

When my parents upped sticks and moved to the Isle of Man, it made our family closer. But it also helped me – if not forced me – to interact with new people. It gave me the skills I needed to be able to talk and listen to others.

There have been times in my life when I have felt confident, and others when I haven't. Usually my issues revolve around weight. I have always been a big guy, and I've always been conscious of it. Even to this day it haunts me. Try finding decent size 14 shoes!

One day when I was 11 years old, I was walking down the steep hill from my parents' restaurant towards the river with a school friend. I was upset because the girl I fancied was far more interested in someone else. He was the fastest runner in school, and those things are so important when you're 11.

'It's all about confidence!' my friend, who was wise beyond his years, declared. 'You need to walk with your head held high, rather than with your chin down and your floppy hair in your face. Being tall is a great thing.'

He had a point.

It's funny what you can remember when you're older. My friend probably doesn't even remember saying these words, but they have stuck with me for the last 20 years. Body language makes all the difference, and I even use this argument in my haircut consultations with clients. Anybody can wear any haircut if they're happy and confident enough to wear it. It's how you enter a room that creates people's opinions of you. Remember, you can only control your own thoughts and actions – no one else's. If you feel confident and happy with yourself, then that is what matters.

I suppose I fell into that "inbetweener" category during secondary school. I was most definitely not a cool, popular kid, but neither was I a geek. I played a lot of sports and loved history and art. My weight fluctuated, and when I was fat people let me know about it. Kids teased me to an extent – and they could definitely be mean – but I wouldn't call it bullying as such. I don't think it was anything other than normal school life. I gave as good as I got too, because boys take the piss out of each other all the time.

It was probably the fact that I was constantly in the "friend zone" with girls that hurt me the most. I was always awkward around them. I put a lot of pressure on myself with regards to my body image. I was always told I was "too nice" too, and I was often discouraged from it. I was also a family boy and I spent most weekends with them, so I missed out on all the underage sex and drinking that was apparently going on down in the park.

I received another good piece of advice from a Sixth-Form girl when I was 15. I was travelling home on the bus from school and feeling desperate for a girlfriend. 'Chin up, Tom,' she told me. 'When you're older, girls will see what a nice guy you are and they will value that, rather than the shallow things girls go for at your age.'

Once again the advice stayed with me for years, even though at the time I thought, *Whatever, I'll be single forever*.

Sadly, once again, and through no fault of my parents, their business in the Isle of Man didn't work out either. They sold the business and decided that we needed another fresh start. And so, in the middle of my GCSEs, we relocated again, this time to Devon.

Now, you may think that moving in the middle of my GCSEs was a terrible idea – lots of people would decide against it. But I personally feel that if I had stayed in the Isle of Man, my grades would have suffered. I felt comfortable in my classes and I had little care for them. I had no real drive or ambition, probably due to limited opportunities on the island.

For a while I thought I wanted to work with animals and I spent a week on work experience at the Manx Wildlife Park. I thoroughly enjoyed it and didn't mind the early morning to travel to the other side of the island to clean up monkey shit. In complete contrast, though, I thoroughly despised the second week, during which I worked in a sports shop. If I learnt one thing there, it was that I never wanted to work in retail.

I had no real desire to study at university either, and I wasn't expected to get phenomenal grades; in fact, the school predicted that I would just scrape by. I was going nowhere pretty fast.

And yet a year or so after we moved to Devon, something changed. I got myself a solid group of friends, one of whom, Ashley, is still a great friend of mine now, 18 years later. (He's also a trustee on the board for The Lions Barber Collective.) The new school meant that I had moved away from the comfort of my friendship group and the expectations of previous teachers, so I, too, had a fresh start.

Looking back, this is when I really began to feel settled, like I belonged somewhere – something we all need and crave. And as a family, we all felt like we were finally home. Everything kind of fitted into place.

So I became the new kid again, and that, in my previous experience, always drew attention. But I decided to concentrate on my exams and took a while to find good friends. This led to me achieving the grades that I needed to do my A Levels – something I never expected previously – and starting to think about the possibility of going to university.

All the moving around and relocating meant that I had become a kind of social chameleon, able to fit into the new classrooms I encountered. I had had some friends that I spent more time with than others, in the way that you do when you're a kid, but I'd never really grown up with anyone and I never had a "core" of best friends, as it were. Maybe I wasn't around long enough?

I don't think it really bothered me too much though. I always managed to make a new group of friends in each school I attended. And as far as I was concerned, I was happy to spend most weekends with my family up until I started doing my A Levels. It wasn't really an active choice; it was just something I enjoyed doing. It wasn't until years later that I realised most other kids were out drinking and smoking in the park and losing their virginities while fumbling around in a crowded room at a sleepover or house party.

I was most definitely a late starter when it came to that side of things. But I wasn't lonely at all – well, no more than the average person (we've all had moments, and sometimes now I actually love being alone, as it is a rarity). In fact, I think all this has made me a stronger person, better adapted for change and unafraid to travel or talk to new people by myself. In fact, if you ask any of my friends now, they will say they hate going on a night out with me because I always ditch them after a few drinks and end up talking to everyone else.

I find meeting new people very interesting, yet I wouldn't say I'm a total extrovert. At times I feel very nervous and out of place, especially if I'm alone in a huge group for the first time. A good example of this is when I went to an awards ceremony for the hair industry recently, which I attended alone. I arrived to see what seemed like thousands of stylists, all standing around in groups or somehow knowing each other. I stood there, scanning the crowd in the square outside the venue, looking for some familiar faces. I eventually found a couple who I spoke to for a brief minute, but then they had to head off and I was alone again. It took me a few drinks before I was comfortable enough to speak to some of the guys who I really looked up to.

So, I suppose it's always depended on the environment. I sometimes have self-confidence issues and struggle with self-doubt when I go to events. Occasionally I doubt that I should even be there; I tell myself I'm out of place, not cool enough or not deserving enough. But we all have those thoughts sometimes, right?

Yes, my weight always posed a problem for me, and even now it's still a struggle. I was unhappy about being overweight, and yet I loved to eat. It never helped that my mum was an amazing chef and I had an extreme sweet tooth, which I blame my grandad for. It's just a shame I didn't get his metabolism! I had the ability to eat sickly stuff when others thought it was too sweet, and I would eat more and more because it tasted good, even if I was full. I never understood it when people would stop eating when they were full. If the food was that good and they could have more, why wouldn't they keep eating? What a major flaw in my mindset!

And because I would eat a lot, I was always offered more. I ended up eating people's leftovers and it became a very bad habit. I would even eat in secret if it was something I wanted. It was a problem that caused me a lot of heartache and sadness. I suppose it is a kind of addiction.

As a kid I hindered myself and put a lot of pressure on myself to be something I thought I should be. In my mind I was convinced that my eating was the reason why I couldn't get a girlfriend, but it never stopped me really.

I see a lot of schoolchildren in my shop, and seeing what they have to go through now – with constant contact not only with their school friends but all others in the area – makes me feel grateful that social media didn't exist back then. The school day ended when I got off that school bus, dragging the double bass (that was the same size as me) out through the doors (through which it just about fit). That was it, school over – well, for that day at least.

I don't look back on my school years with regret or pain. It was just school, a part of my life that I enjoyed. I had good and bad days, and it affected my mental health in different ways. But it served the purpose of education and social interaction. There are a lot of things that could have been better, but also many things could have been worse.

My school days weren't "the happiest years of my life" as we so often hear. I find this saying so upsetting – shouldn't we all try to be happy with the things we have now, rather than looking back sadly at the "good old days"?

CHAPTER 4

HARDCORE KID ALEX

And so during my A Levels, I started to go out and interact with more people. I gained more confidence and even started to draw attention from the opposite sex, something I had longed for throughout my school life with no success.

To be honest, I'm still not sure if this wasn't only down to the self-belief that only three cans of Red Stripe could give me. And maybe the girls drank Red Stripe or Mad Dog 20/20 too, before they entered the club. (Although I must say that more often than not we would all meet at the steps of the multi-storey car park in the centre of town. How classy those years were!)

Either way, my self-confidence grew whenever I went out. I also lost my excess weight and became part of a gang that went to the local rock club and the pub every weekend. It almost felt like a family, and that bubble was my world. The rock club – called The Hideaway – was everything back then. We hid away from all the worries of Sixth Form and anything else in that place. It was dark and dingy, down an alley behind the McDonald's in Torquay. We would hang out outside the club before and after it was open, with a multi-storey car park looming over us. In fact, I think we spent just as much time in that concrete structure as we did in the club. I can remember sitting there on the stairs, mostly talking shit and drinking a big bottle of WKD. Someone would come running out to tell us that the DJ, Big Nick or Glen, was playing the song we had requested. We'd drop everything – well, we'd place our glass bottles down carefully so as not to waste any booze – and run inside to start our own little mosh pit. We'd listen to the latest song from System of a Down or Papa Roach, or a classic from the likes of Pantera or Rob Zombie.

I actually found a tape recently from the time that I took my parents' video camera to the club. I told them I was going to film my friend's puppies – it even has a sticker on the tape saying "Puppies!" I managed to get it digitalised and share it with everyone who used to go there. I haven't even managed to watch it all yet – it'll be way too cringey. The few minutes I have watched took me back to a time when there wasn't any social media and no one had camera phones. What happened on that night out stayed there. It's pretty crazy to think about, now that we document *everything*. You cannot get away with anything today. I can pretty comfortably bet that everyone reading this – everyone who has been drunk on a night out since the invention of the camera phone – has had a photo or video taken of themselves on someone else's phone that they hate.

It's not a great thing to wake up with a sore head, only to find you're tagged in a video of you streaking along the beach and that it's been posted on all social media platforms. (Just for the record, that never happened. Well, there's no video evidence, anyway.)

All of a sudden I had a lot of female attention. Maybe it was too much. I was spoilt for choice after being starved of it. It just felt so amazing to feel desired after I'd chased that feeling for so long. My own insecurities took over, and I felt shocked whenever anyone showed me any interest. I literally couldn't resist it. I was like a kid in a sweet shop, and with my sweet tooth it was dangerous! I just wanted to have my cake and it too (again, with the cake and eating!).

God knows why I put myself through the stress of trying to manage more than one girl at any time. It certainly wasn't good for me, just as it wasn't good for them. But back in those early days of going to the rock club, it was almost innocent. It was also kind of expected in my circle for guys to be like that at the time. Maybe it's a kind of macho thing to prove a point or fight an insecurity, to confirm that you're desirable, needed, or attractive. I expect each of us had our reasoning behind this kind of behaviour.

In fact, the more I acted that way, the more girls paid interest, and personally I think this is still the case, especially when younger. I see it a lot through work and I have often had conversations with guys in the chair about the pressure of multiple lovers. And a fair few have sat in my chair and told me that all they want is a long-term steady relationship, yet their friends that play the field get all the girls and don't treat them right. It's possibly even worse now, with the likes of dating apps like Tinder, which have made relationships even more throwaway than ever.

Seeing the way younger clients treat relationships is unreal. I see both men and women consistently setting up three or four dates for one weekend, and it all seems to be normal. I wonder where it'll lead?

I was definitely not a model boyfriend, and I went from girl to girl like a magpie with shiny objects. I couldn't resist that attention, and I had a lot of fun with it. I had become one of the lads that I'd hated so much in school for taking advantage of girls. I was in my own little world and I definitely hurt some people along the way.

But I didn't see it. I was so insular that I wasn't even really aware that I was hurting other people (or even that I *could* hurt others). I was just riding the wave while it lasted, and it lasted quite some time. I did settle down a few times and had long-term girlfriends, but my head always got turned in the end. I loved the chase. I don't think I was ever malicious, and I never set out to hurt anyone. I always felt such terrible guilt if I ever did cheat on a girl, and I was always fearful of hurting them if they ever found out. It's such a ridiculous thing to put yourself through, let alone another person.

But, as it does, karma came back to bite me. After a lot of years, I had a girl from my past contact me. In the past I had often looked back at our relationship with regret for messing it all up. At first I was shocked when she told me she wanted to meet, but I decided I should. I had all sorts of things going through my head. I kind of saw her as "the one who got away", although it was me who had fucked up at the time. I went and met her and she asked me why I had done all those things I'd done to her years ago when we were teenagers.

I didn't have an answer. I didn't know. All I could tell her was that I hadn't set out to hurt her. I'd been selfish, and I'd never even thought that I would have such an effect on someone. Now, however, the guilt was horrendous. I felt awful that it had affected her so much. I felt awful that she wanted to know why it had happened, and I couldn't give her any better answer than 'I was young' and 'I couldn't resist'.

It feels a bit moronic that I wasn't aware of how much messing someone about could hurt someone else. It wasn't a personal attack on them, and it wasn't a comment on anything they had done, but I have learnt an important lesson: never underestimate your actions and how they can affect others.

I continued to behave in this way occasionally for a while. As I got older, doing these things got easier because the tech became more advanced. With text messaging and the internet, I suddenly had the ability to contact more people – 24 / 7. Plus, I'd got a gym membership and I was slimmer and fitter than ever before. I had confidence and more disposable income with which to buy stylish clothing and tattoos.

The rock club was the hub of my social life, and it was all that was important to me. My love for music grew and grew, and it became the main thing in my life. I spent all of my time and money on it, and all my friends revolved around it. Being into punk music, I gravitated towards some of the punk guys and I spent a fair bit of time with the local bands and those who were at their gigs. Saying that, the punks did hang out with the guys who were into metal and everything in between. My eclectic taste in music meant that I had friends who were solely metalheads too. Some of my friends were more straight-edge, hardcore kids and some were old-school, heavy-drinking, drug-taking punks. It meant that when we were out on the town, there were very few people I didn't know.

One weekend a guy noticed an F-Minus band shirt I was wearing. He came up to me and, very enthusiastically, he started discussing their latest release and the fact that they were touring. He mentioned that they would be playing at a local live music venue – The Cavern – in Exeter, and that we should go and see them. With that, the tickets were bought and the date marked off. On the day we all piled into a friend's car (it was small and his first car!) and travelled up to see the band. I felt kind of privileged to be in on that. It was like being part of an exclusive group, you know? Like I had made it with the cool kids.

In that moment I felt like I belonged. It's a great feeling, especially when you've found those people who, in your perception, are totally into the same things as you. I mean, we were into obscure, small-time hardcore punk that no one else listens to! I just suppose it was one of those moments when everything feels right in the world. You know, those moments that come and go. One day everything is right in the world and you're making all the right decisions with the right people. Next thing you know, you see something online or receive an email or text and you're questioning your decisions and worry about what direction to take. That's normal, right?

It's amazing how something like a band shirt can instantly unite people, especially if the band is obscure. It's different now that rock T-shirts are available in high-street stores and worn as fashion items. Asking someone about a T-shirt now can often be answered with a blank stare.

I also happened to be in a screamo band, and I really enjoyed the success we had locally. The band was called Beneath Cutting Lies and there were five of us in total. We used to practise in a church hall every Sunday. It was a blast! We thought we were in with a chance of making it big (which to us meant being signed to an indie label and supporting some of the Californian bands we loved so much) but playing The Townhouse pub and packing it out still felt brilliant. At one gig everyone left after we played and didn't stay around for the next acts. Looking back I feel a little bit sorry for those bands, but at the time I was like, 'Wow! People came to see us!'

(I decided to celebrate that with a crate of banana bread beer. Jesus, I haven't thought about that in a while. Do they even still make that stuff?)

That was the first time I can really remember hanging out with Hardcore Kid Alex. My girlfriend at the time – who didn't really live in our Townhouse / Hideaway bubble – gave him the name. He listened to hardcore music, although not exclusively, and he dressed like a "hardcore kid". Hardcore is a subgenre of punk music (Google Black Flag, Terror, Misfits, or Minor Threat) and it was popular within our social circle at the time. I'm a little uncertain if his wardrobe – or mine, for that matter – contained any colour other than black.

On the first evening I met him, I learnt that Alex not only had impeccable taste in music and was quite opinionated, but he was also a pro-wrestling (not sports entertainment) fan. There aren't a lot of wrestling fans about, so when wrestling fans meet one another we stick together. Not many people go about shouting how much they love watching two men in pants, fighting each other in a choreographed battle with a pre-determined outcome – especially for the fear of those 'You do know it's fake?' comments.

Alex and I knew that wrestling was "fake", but it is an art form that is there solely for the entertainment of the viewer. The fact that we both knew that is one of the many reasons we were friends.

Wrestling has always been a strong and important bonding feature within my friendship circles, and it still is. I dread to think how many hours of it I've watched, but it's brought me close to a lot people. Wrestling seemed to be a bit of a guilty pleasure of ours; it's something we kept a secret, and it created a bit of unity between us all. Maybe others didn't get it, but we loved it. If you know, you know!

Alex also introduced me to CZW (combat zone wrestling), an extreme hardcore company (to give you an idea of what it's like, they hold events such as the annual "Tournament of Death"). Around this time I was living in a flat with my best mate Ash above a pub on Torquay Harbour, and we'd spend hours watching DVDs of Japanese wrestling together. We had to have it turned up loud because of the sound of seagulls nesting on our flat! (Looking back, I don't know why we bothered, because all the commentary was in Japanese. I certainly don't know any, and I am pretty sure Alex didn't either, although we definitely spent enough time watching it that we might have picked up a few words.)

Our friendship was mostly centred around a hub of music and wrestling. We would most often see each other out on the town rather than plan to go out together, but whenever I saw him we'd end up spending a fair bit of time together. Our passions were niche and, like most other young guys, we spent a lot of time talking about what excited us. We would focus on that and only that, only switching it up when one of us broke up with a girl, or fell out with a friend, or went through some other emotionally charged event. Fuelled by alcohol on a night out, we'd pour our hearts out on the fire escape steps outside The Townhouse or down on the concrete steps at Breakwater beach.

Alex was a fun guy. He was always in the middle of it all. He had his finger on the pulse when it came to anything new and innovative in live music or wrestling, and we were always there together on the scene. I learnt a lot from him. He had a great group of friends and I was lucky to be considered one of them.

When it came to deciding whether I wanted to go to university, I realised that education and academia were no longer for me, despite the fact that I had managed to pass all my A Levels – even geography, which I hated. (I didn't even really want to do geography. I hadn't studied it at GCSE level. I wanted to go into marine biology, but my sciences weren't good enough. So, when the teacher who interviewed me found out that I liked sport, he suggested that I do PE – which is basically bloody biology and I couldn't do that either – and geography, because apparently that's good for the leisure industry. I turned up to my first class and who was the teacher? The teacher who had interviewed me! Maybe he needed more people in his class? God knows, but I found it dull because he wasn't the most charismatic of my teachers.)

It was becoming hard work to keep up on studying. Not only was I having fun and enjoying a great social life – very often the main focal point of your life when you're 18 – but I just knew I didn't really want to do it anymore. And if I went to university, I knew I would only be going there to watch live music, drink, chase women, and use my student loan to get tattoos. Probably not a wise choice. And so I made the decision to tread another path instead. But what would I do? Knowing that I wasn't going to go to university was a good thing, but I needed another plan.

Well, although the answer was staring me in the face, I didn't see it until my mum mentioned it.

'Hairdressing!' she said to me. 'Why don't you do hairdressing?'

How the hell hadn't I thought of that? It made perfect sense! I coloured my own hair and cut it nearly every week – I had even been cutting a lot of my friends' hair in my spare time! It also bamboozled me that no one else had ever mentioned it to me as a possibility, given my ever-changing head of hair. The teachers at my Sixth Form would always comment on my changing hairstyle every couple of weeks. How confusing then that none of them had said to me, 'Why don't you do hairdressing?' when I came to them struggling for ideas! It was almost as though there wasn't another option for me – I had done my A Levels and my predicted grades were good enough, so why wouldn't I go to university?

My mum wanted to be a hairdresser when she was younger but had been advised to go into banking as a more stable job with a better income, but this definitely wasn't a "parent living their dream through their child" kind of deal. She had never mentioned it to me before, but as soon as she did, something clicked. The idea felt right straightaway. I looked at my hair in the mirror, styling it, thinking, *this is meant to be*. I had some clarity on my future.

So that was decided: I was going to try to get into hairdressing. I went back to school, excited to tell all of my teachers that I had made a decision: the decision that I wasn't going to fill in my UCAS form, but look at a career in the hair industry instead.

The response wasn't what I expected. I was told by all of my teachers –all except my sociology teacher, who was a feminist lesbian and thought it was fantastic that a straight male was giving up the opportunity to go to university and becoming a hairdresser instead – that it was a disappointing decision. They told me I should achieve the grades to go to uni and put all my focus into that during the last term of my A Levels.

It really knocked me back. I had found what I wanted to do, and it was almost soul destroying for them to pretty much shoot me down straight off the bat.

Now, I don't know if they didn't like the idea of me going into the hair industry because it was "beneath" an A Level student, or because they needed as many of their students to go to university as possible in order to make their statistics look good and therefore keep their funding. But either way, it was hard to take. Their negativity surrounded and overwhelmed me, and it seemed to come from all directions, which shocked me to no end. I believed I'd made a really positive decision, and I didn't want them to make me doubt what I actually wanted.

And although I can't remember feeling angry at the time, looking back now I find it unbelievable that those teachers weren't supportive of a student who was making a decision based on what he wanted to do and enjoyed doing. Surely that is something we are taught from day one? How does the saying go? 'If you can do a job you love, then you will never work a day in your life', or something to that effect?

I had found my dream career path. I was just focused on what I wanted to do. I felt like I had a direction, instead of just meandering through further education and being uncertain of my path. Thankfully I didn't feel like I was letting anyone down. I was 100 per cent behind this choice and there was no doubt in my mind that the hair industry was the right choice for me, my personality, and my creative mind. I was moving in the right direction.

The funny thing is that when I started at Toni & Guy (a job I managed to secure by volunteering there every Saturday for the last 10 weeks of school), female assistants all seemed to share the same point of view as my teachers.

'What are you doing here?' they'd ask me, repeatedly. 'I wish I'd worked harder at school so I could have gone to university.'

Others had different reactions. For example, when I told my friends at school, there were a lot of the classic, predictable questions. 'Oh, you're going to be a hairdresser? Are you gay?' Surprisingly, though, this didn't bother me. I never really worried about that when I considered joining the industry. Maybe it's because I was always comfortable with my sexuality. Besides, I always just thought that my friends were joking around, although I can see now why people would think it was a negative thing. Having said that, every time my friends came back from university during school breaks, they always wanted to meet me from work – and I'm pretty sure it had something to do with the 15 or so female hairdressers that worked with me. It was pretty funny, actually, when they realised that I – a straight, male hairdresser – was spending pretty much all my time with the opposite sex. It made quite a few of my friends quite jealous!

I now know that deciding to leave school and jump into the hair industry was the best decision I could have ever made, especially because, as I'm writing this, I'm currently on my way to the Hawaiian island of Maui to work for a week. There's not that many jobs that give you these kinds of opportunities while doing something that you enjoy so much.

CHAPTER 5

THE GOOD SAMARITAN

I had found a job with one of the largest companies in the hair industry, one with an incredible reputation.

And yet, it was at this point in my life that things got hard.

I wasn't any more nervous than is "normal" for an 18-year-old starting a new job. I wasn't lying awake at night, worrying or panicking about problems that might or might not happen. I think that came a lot later in life. I was pretty confident about things like this; after all, moving to new places, meeting new people, and experiencing new situations had been the norm for me since I was young, what with all the relocating I had done with my family.

The problem was that the pull of university had taken all of my friends away from me. I think this is probably true of people in most small seaside towns, but there wasn't a huge number of the population that fit into the 18–21 category, and even fewer who were in the "alternative" bracket.

I felt incredibly alone.

Some nights I would come home from work and go up to my room, up in the attic of the quaint little cottage we lived in at the time, and sit on my bed. I would go through my phone and look through my numbers and text messages. I realised that everyone was scattered around the country at different universities, and I no longer had any friends at home. I would just lie there on my bed crying, feeling very lonely.

Now that I think about it, there were obviously still some people around, but this was back in the days when you could only store 10 texts at a time on your phone and you had to be very careful about which ones you saved. Deciding what messages you could delete so that you could receive some more was very difficult.

One night I realised that everyone who had sent me the last 10 text messages had all gone.

It was a difficult time. The group that had disbanded and left had been pretty tight-knit. We'd spent most of our time together discussing, watching, and listening to music. And now everyone who had lived in the same small town as me had gone. What a big moment in my young life.

I had moved schools many times in the past, always leaving everyone behind and moving on to the next group of people. But this time it was everyone else who had moved on – and it was me who was left behind.

These feelings would hit me hardest when I was alone in the evenings. I didn't really talk about them because I knew there wasn't anything wrong with me. I just considered this completely normal, which it is, isn't it? Having your entire friendship group move away *would* make you feel a bit shit, right?

I just had to do what I had managed to do before with relative ease: move into another group of people and make more of the company around me – those who previously I'd only regarded as recognisable faces on a night out.

Things did slowly improve. As time passed, I really started to enjoy my role at Toni & Guy. Being in a social business such as hairdressing meant that I met loads of people every day and was invited to lots of events, parties, and nights out. That meant that I started to spend less time alone, and when I did, I had the security of knowing that it was my choice, and if I wanted to meet someone or go somewhere, I could call a friend and have the company if I wanted it.

It was definitely a defining moment in my life. All of my previous friends had been in my year at school or maybe in the year above or below. But as soon as I went into the world of full-time work, my friendship group evolved rapidly and I was exposed to a much wider variety of people. Within my new circle of friends there was an age range from 16 to 60+.

I was really lucky to have some great teachers and role models who taught me a lot about life as well as hair – I owe a lot of that to my colleagues Tim, Barrie, Phil, and John. They all worked with me at Toni & Guy and were the inspiration for many of my hair industry dreams; they moulded me into the hair professional that I am today.

I spent a lot of time with these guys outside of work as well as in the salon, and I was keen to listen to their stories and history. They had all done a lot in the industry and they kept me motivated. I would often finish work and go to one of the nearby pubs with one of them and carry on talking about hair for hours. And even though they were all so different from one another, their passion for the hair industry let me know that I had made the right decision.

Barrie Radford was a stylist who had an eye for cutting the latest styles and always pushing the boundaries. He taught me to forget that "the box" existed. We'd go out into Torquay at the weekends and if I stayed at his place (I lived with my parents in Brixham at the time – it was £20 for a taxi ride or the equivalent of another two rounds of drinks. Guess which option won?) we would stay up into the early hours discussing hair and upcoming trends. The song 'Don't Stop Me Now' by Queen will always remind me of him.

Tim Mileham had been part of the Toni & Guy artistic team and as a result he'd done a lot of huge shows. One day, while I was sitting at the salon revising my step-by-steps, I saw him on the Toni & Guy channel on the TV, working on this big stage.

What the ...?! I thought, blinking up at the screen. *That's Tim! You can really go and do this sort of thing? You can really go onstage and do hair in front of crowds of people?*

That gave me my first bit of inspiration for becoming a session stylist, and now it's something I do all the time. Tim opened my eyes to that possibility, giving me so much confidence and believing in my capability from day one.

John Mudie took over as manager at Toni & Guy, and he always looked after me. I'd spend a lot of time with him discussing the hair industry. He was the best person I have ever worked with at customer service and he took the time to explain its significance. He taught me that it isn't all about the haircut; the service, experience, and the bond between client and stylist is just as important, if not more. And his blowdrying skills were something to be envious of. Because of this, his column was jam-packed all day, every day.

When John broke his leg, a man called Phil Collins came from head office to manage the salon. He had a wealth of knowledge and experience in London with both Toni&Guy and TIGI hair products. It was like he was from another world compared to Torquay but we got on straightaway. I am still in close contact with Phil and I firmly believe that without his knowledge and support I would not have had the confidence to look beyond Devon as a hair professional.

One night when I was 18, the team all went out for a meal at a huge table at Pizza Express. It was my boss's birthday and he was turning 30 years old. *Jesus, that is so grown-up*, I thought to myself as I sat there, drinking wine. *This is all so mature.* In all honesty, I think the influence of all those people of different ages and tastes helped me grow a lot in a short period of time. It became especially noticeable when some of the guys would return from university and I began to find them immature. It was as if I had started to outgrow them.

There's no doubt that the job brought me out of myself. I started to go out at the weekends with the girls from the team and their boyfriends. They often went to drum and bass raves, where I would stand out like a sore thumb – standing at 6ft 3in with a pink mohawk, leather jacket, ripped bleached jeans, and my Doc Martens, I wasn't exactly the average raver!

Fears of being picked out and ridiculed for my appearance would fly around my mind.

What if I don't get accepted because I'm a punk at a rave?

What if their friends don't wanna hang out and I'm left alone at the club?

Will they understand that I just wanna have a good night like them?

Will they think I'm at the wrong club?

Will I get shunned?

When I walked the streets, I would often get shouted at or abused by people in passing cars just because of the way I looked. Whether I was sporting a pink mohawk, rockabilly quiff, pompadour, or long hair, I had the attire to go with it. I can remember being called Elvis when I had my pompadour the first time around – like it was a bad thing! This is the haircut that half the population now sports! Strange how fashion and trends change opinions.

Fortunately, my worries over being judged or being the butt of everyone's jokes at the raves couldn't have been further from the truth. Everyone was incredibly welcoming, and more than anything they were intrigued about how I was dressed and how my hair stood up on end all night.

I guess if you take the amount of ecstasy that most of those guys in the club would have on a night out, then there's not a lot of room for anger – only love! It meant that those I would normally be scared of when walking down the street would actually come up to me, ask questions, and speak to me on their level. So it wasn't all bad.

This kind of experience greatly improved my confidence, and I started finding the strength to go out by myself and go to the local alternative clubs and pubs. I got involved in that scene often by turning up by myself, but I didn't care anymore. Besides, there were a lot of familiar faces.

It was always fun whenever there was an opportunity to go to a festival with everyone. I absolutely loved festivals. There would always be a big group of us from all the pubs and clubs – in fact, there were so many of us that by the time we'd set up camp it would look as though we'd created our own little mini-Devon!

My first festival was Reading festival in 2001. It blew me away. I stayed up all night completely sober, just walking the miles and miles of camp sites, meeting new people and talking about music for hours. It was amazing. The Download festival at Donnington, however – the home of heavy metal – was different. Some of my favourite bands were playing and I was feeling more confident and content in myself. Everything seemed awesome and I had a new, stable group of friends, so the decision to go was a total no-brainer.

Then, out of nowhere, my grandad died. It was totally unexpected. He was making his way up to bed one night and he just dropped dead.

I received the call while I was at work behind the bar in the pub I lived above at the time (I had started to work a few shifts there to pay the rent). I was in shock and I had to stop working. The landlord, who was Ashley's mum and like a second mother to me) got me a brandy and comforted me. Grandad had owned a pub before I was born, and I'd heard all sorts of stories about that, so on reflection it seems kind of fitting that I was standing behind a bar when I was told that he was gone.

Grandad Billy was the first person I had ever lost, and it hit me really hard. I loved him. I remember lying in bed when I was young, thinking, I don't want my grandparents to die. And even though their deaths were way in the future at that point (not that you ever know when people will die), I still worried about it. I was pretty young, and I feared the deaths of my family.

And now it had happened – I'd lost him.

Admittedly, on top of all this shock, I did think, *Shit, I can't go to Download festival now, not now that we've lost Grandad Billy*. It's a silly thing to think about really, but I was young and had been looking forward to attending such a big event with my friends. But it was okay. I talked to my mum – who was obviously devastated to have lost her dad – and she convinced me to go to Download and try to enjoy myself, as Billy would've wanted me to.

I still wasn't sure it was the right thing to do. I felt guilty about having fun when I maybe shouldn't have done. I should have just felt sad, right?

But in the end, Download was the perfect excuse to drink away my sorrows. I think I pretty much drank from before my tent was up until I fell asleep on the last night.

Something amazing happened that night as I walked through the "village". The village is basically where the official club tent and all the stalls and funfair are located. It's a crazy place if I'm honest, and it has a Mad Max / apocalyptic kind of feel. Everyone feels a bit hazy because they're all intoxicated and feeling a little bit rough around the edges. When I was there you could still have open fires, so there were tents surrounded by campfire smoke, cigarette smoke, and the smell of dirt, alcohol, Portaloos, and sweat.

Our funds were low as we made our way through the crowd, and we were hungry. 'Samaritans always have a tent, and their food is well cheap,' said one of the gang.

'Yeah, it's like 10p for soup,' someone else chipped in.

That decided it. We went to find the Samaritans' tent, which was very basic, and they were right – it was something like 20p for a cup of soup and a roll. *Unbelievable*, I thought. What a find that was!

As my very blurry memory recalls, one of the Samaritan guys asked me, 'So, buddy, how are you? Enjoying the festival?'

I was pretty drunk at the time, and I answered him politely with the most common of answers, the type you'll get out of most people when you ask them if they are okay.

'Yeah, I'm alright mate,' I replied.

But then something important happened. He asked me, 'You sure? You can tell me anything, you know. That's what we're trained to do – listen.'

That's all he did. He made himself available to me, inviting me to tell him what I was feeling and let out what I needed. After a moment I sobered up, and that's when losing my grandad really hit me. I told the guy everything.

Poor bloke, I thought. *I bet he wishes he'd never asked now*. But I went on anyway, going back to all the lovely memories I had, telling him that Billy was the first person I'd lost and how I could never have been prepared for it. I told him I was worried for my nan and mum. I told him that my grandad was a brilliant man, the head of the family, strong and ready to help solve any problems. I'd looked up to him and aspired to be like him. I even told him about the littlest things, like how we'd called custard creams "Grandad Billy biscuits" because he'd always had them with his tea.

And finally, I told him about how I felt about how I'd never see my grandad again.

Even though there were 80,000 people at Download festival, for a short while it felt like it was only me and the wonderful Samaritan in that field.

I never got to thank him, really. I mean, I thanked him as I left the tent and ventured back into the wild world of the campsite, but I wish I'd had the chance to thank him again properly. That guy really made a difference to me, and all he did was listen. It was such a powerful thing, and it lifted a huge weight off me.

When I got back from the festival we had to get through the funeral. It was intense. At first I was asked to carry the coffin into the church, but I couldn't do it. I just couldn't do it. It meant saying goodbye forever.

When we got inside, the church was full – so full that some people had to stand up at the back, and this wasn't a small church. I knew my grandad had been popular and had had his fingers in all sorts of pies, but I never realised that he'd touched this many people's lives. The church was packed considering it was a funeral for a 76-year-old, and that made me proud to be his grandson.

When we headed over to the crematorium, I had another opportunity to carry the coffin. I knew that I couldn't miss it this time; it was my last chance to hold him and say goodbye. So I stepped up and took him onto my shoulder.

It was so heavy and uncomfortable on my shoulder. *What if I walk too fast?* I worried. *What if I drop it?* But in the end, I didn't care. I knew he was there right next to me for one last time, just on the other side of that wood. I spoke to him all the way down the aisle. It was difficult, but I thank him still for everything he has done.

The wake was amazing. It was such a high after a terrible low. I saw all of his family members who I hadn't seen since I was a small child. It was a lovely sunny day and all the grandkids were in the hotel's gardens. They had a DVD playing on a big drop-down screen, showing the game where England won the Ashes. Everyone shared stories about great times with Grandad Billy, discussing his kind gestures, hard work, and funny stories.

Mum told us all about the time that she and Dad needed some stairs leading down from a first-floor fire escape, and they told

Grandad Billy about it. And so then, one day, he just turned up with some stairs for them. No one knew where they were from! It gave me a mental image of someone just going out to have a cigarette on the fire escape on their lunchbreak one day, opening the door and realising that their stairs weren't there. Imagine the look on their face.

I mean, how the hell do you even transport a set of metal stairs?

I suppose it's difficult when you're 18 and you're too old to want to spend time with the other children, but there's also a generation gap between you and the adults who are all parents and grandparents. But that day I had a pint of Guinness for the first time ever, and having a pint with my relatives kind of made me feel like a grown-up.

It was almost like a passing of the torch, a transition into becoming one of the "adults" in the family rather than one of the kids.

CHAPTER 6

TURNING DOWN
A BAD DEAL

For a long time, music was my first love. It was my dream and my passion. Hair was my job, but I dreamt of being a rock star and playing our songs onstage, with people singing the lyrics back to us. Beneath Cutting Lies had broken up when some of the band members went to uni, so I became the fake-blood-spitting, face paint-wearing frontman of a new "deathcore" or "metalcore" band, No Such Thing As A King. It took up pretty much all my spare time, if I'm honest.

We practised on Wednesday evenings and all day on Sundays. We even had a room of our own to practise in and spent a lot of time in there, much to the despair of the band members' girlfriends at the time. It was funny really, because girls liked the fact that we were in a band, but hated that we had to practise and travel to play shows. It was a big issue for more than one band member! And when we weren't playing or practising, we were managing our MySpace account, writing lyrics, or recording.

Luckily the original guitarist, a guy name Jay, was amazingly gifted when it came to sound. He could seriously play, but he could also record, mix, and master. This led to us recording an EP with him pretty quickly. Our stand-out style made us pretty popular in the local scene. It was great fun.

Once we had our logo and EP done, it was time to push ourselves out there and realise our dream of becoming rock stars. Now we had to put in the hours. I can remember sitting at my computer and copying our songs onto CD after CD, sending them out relentlessly to record labels. I messaged record labels online too. My excitement was real – like a-kid-on-Christmas-Eve real. It's the kind of excitement that keeps you awake at night. You don't have that feeling very often as an adult. With every message or CD I sent out, I honestly believed I would get something. I felt we were that good.

I think the original line-up had huge potential to become a successful band. We had a good look for the time, a unique sound, and catchy songs. That's not often the case with heavier genres of metal. It seemed like a great combination. However, after two members left and we found their replacements (twin brothers who played bass and guitar and were also awesome at what they did) we became heavier in style. It seemed that we lost the uniqueness that we had before.

It was still all very exciting at this point, though, and we had some great songs. We even made a video, which is still out there on YouTube somewhere. We played some great shows supporting some brilliant bands. The extreme nature of my stage presence – the face paint, the spitting fake blood, and climbing on anything I could – combined with some unruly behaviour from some of the band members meant that we did get banned from a few venues. But hey, we saw that as a good thing. At least we had impact! People had an opinion about us, both good and bad. And there's nothing worse than people not caring at all.

Maybe we should have played on that a bit more at the time. We had a few offers from record labels over the time we played together, but we didn't sign any.

One in particular stands out for me. We received a message back from the independent record label, saying that the head of the company had listened to us and loved what he'd heard.

He also loved our name and our logo. He invited us to meet him at this house where their studio was. Now, if there had been a contract there and then to sign, I would have signed it in a heartbeat. In my head, I was about to be given everything I had ever wanted. We were going to be featured in magazines, playing to crowds of people who knew our songs. We were going to have our CDs on the shelves (that was the most common way to buy music then) and our own merchandise. We were going to tour the world!

First, we had to convince the rest of the band to go up and see this guy. We had to drive to Norwich – which, if you live in the Southwest, is pretty much the furthest you can drive without heading to Scotland. So one day we all piled into one car and set off. It started out with excitement, and we joked on the way up about what we would do if the postcode we were following in the sat-nav was just his own road and nothing else. But after hours and hours of driving in a small Ford full of five fully grown blokes, the excitement died off and the discomfort set in.

When we arrived, we realised that the postcode was, in fact, for a private lane, down which there was a huge country house with land and outbuildings hidden away from the main road. He really did have his own road! Wow!

As we drove down the lane he spotted us through the huge bay window of his office.

'Shit! He's seen us!' one of the guys shouted.

We'd planned it all out in the car: we'd arrive and get out, take a stroll, and freshen up. Those who smoked would have a cigarette and we'd all decide on where we stood on any contract discussions. Well, that all went out the window when he saw us and we had to go straight in!

He came out to meet us and took us through to his office, which was full of recording equipment. According to our guitarist, who had done all of our previous recordings, it was worth tens of thousands of pounds. As we all sat there looking at him from across his desk, all I could think was, *I've made it. We're going to sign our contract today, and I'm going to be the frontman of a signed metal band!*

I don't think I was listening closely enough to anything he had to say really, except that we would have a multi-album deal, merchandise designed by his designer – who would also do our album artwork – and we would record our songs there at his studio on site. And we'd stay in one of the big outbuildings he'd had converted.

I was in. I would have done it right there and then. And I think most of the other guys would have too.

However, the bassist at the time was the sensible one. He had a brother who worked in law, and so he suggested that we take the contract to him and let him look at it. Without everyone's signatures we couldn't do anything, so that was what we decided to do. We had to get straight back in the car and drive for another six or seven hours back home.

That journey wasn't so exciting, but I can't recall anyone being angry that our bandmate wanted his brother to look over the contract. I think that was the best, most mature decision we made. I can't imagine how many groups of young lads just sign anything pushed under their noses with the offer of becoming a signed artist.

A few days went by and we were all eager to find out his brother's thoughts. I remember us all nagging him quite a lot, but in our opinion it wasn't too much – this could have been our future. The guy from the record label was also keen to know our decision, and he messaged us a lot. It made me think positively, that maybe he saw something in us. But the news came back negative on the contract and my heart sank.

After the initial heartbreak, I listened properly to the reasons as to why we shouldn't take the deal. I realised pretty quickly that it was a very poor deal for us, one that would most likely see us ending up in financial trouble and / or stuck in a terrible deal we had no way of getting out of. We'd have had to put another four albums together in order to fulfil our side of the contract, and we'd have been in a lot of debt.

Turning it down was the best thing that could have happened really, even though at the time all I wanted was to be in a signed band. I'd put all my energy into it and wanted to live that stereotypical rock star lifestyle, but I thank my bandmate's brother eternally for helping us avoid a bad deal.

CHAPTER 7

PAUSE FOR THOUGHT: GOALS

Surely goals are something we all have, or at least something we should all have?

At work, I am lucky enough to meet and talk to many people of all ages and backgrounds on a daily basis. I have developed into a kind of social chameleon, adapting to whoever I am with by listening to and learning from them.

However, it came to my surprise that, when conversing with a lot of people about goals and plans for the upcoming year, the vast majority seemed to have none at all – nor had they even considered it. My Action Day Planner states that up to 97 per cent of people do not set goals, which seems like too many. One person who I have known for some time seemed to have little motivation and no vision into their own future at all, other than the day-to-day routine of going to work at a job they didn't like, to receive a wage they weren't happy with, and nowhere to progress within their current organisation.

When I asked about their aspirations and goals, they didn't seem to have any.

When I asked, 'What is your dream? No matter how crazy it is, what would you love to do?' there was a silence.

Then they replied, 'That's quite hard to think about, when you're actually asked.'

This made me feel devastated. A young person of 21 didn't seem to have a dream, let alone a goal or even a resolution.

'What are your interests, hobbies, or loves? You could do something to do with any of them. Today we are so connected globally, you could start a niche business in *your* interest, from your own bedroom!' I said.

When he replied, 'I'd never thought about it like that before,' I hoped I might have sparked something in him.

We are so lucky to live in a world today where we have so many opportunities that the generations before us didn't have. I believe goal-setting can get you en route to achieving your dreams.

Decide what you want. This is your direction. Set yourself goals in order to reach your destination, and you may be surprised how quickly you achieve each one.

I'm looking forward to seeing this particular client for their next appointment.

CHAPTER 8

NEW OPPORTUNITIES

When the band finally split up, I realised how much I actually loved doing hair and what a great job I had. At this point I'd been in the industry for nearly 10 years – after the Toni & Guy branch had closed down, I'd got a job at a salon that was run by a girl who'd gone through her apprenticeship alongside me. We'd got to know each other throughout the entirety of our careers. We were very good friends, qualifying together at Manchester Toni & Guy academy. I'd even spent my 21st birthday with her on a train to the academy, and we'd had a dinner together at the Hard Rock Café. I remember her buying me a Cadbury's Creme Egg as a present on the train. Strange how I remember that, as I couldn't even tell you anything else I had that year for a birthday gift!

My job didn't feel like work, and as I'd been in the industry for nearly a decade, I had a loyal clientele. And so I spent a couple more years after the band split up just concentrating on my career. During this time I devoted a lot more time to my own skills, passion, and work ethic, being the first to arrive and last to leave and proving my value with each passing day.

And so, eventually, I felt like I was in a position to start my own salon. I had built up a reasonable reputation in the area over that time and I finally felt focused.

I had spent many years chasing a dream – the dream of travelling the world and doing something I loved. And I knew, deep down, that I could do that with hair, because I'd seen Tim doing it when working at Toni & Guy. I'd since watched all the videos of these huge international hair or fashion shows and I'd attended big events, so I knew it was possible. But I thought it was only possible if I lived in London, and there was no way I would have left Devon for the busier, crowded urban lifestyle.

And so with the help of my parents – who supported me financially, physically, and mentally – I started the journey of setting up Tom Chapman Hair Design. Leaving my previous salon – where I was a self-employed stylist – was an incredibly hard thing to do, as I had been with them for seven years. But I needed to further my career and take this opportunity to have the creative freedom I desired. I wanted the ability to make some decisions for myself.

I was very stressed about telling my friend I was going to leave, and I put it off for a while for fear of her reaction and the worry of upsetting and letting the team down. It played on me every day, but I knew deep down I was doing something to better my life and I hoped that she and her parents – who had helped her with the development of her business – would understand. They'd created this opportunity for their daughter and so I knew it was a big deal for them.

When I did pluck up the courage to tell them about six weeks before I started my own business, they were not happy at all and I was told I had to leave the next day. This was heartbreaking and upsetting, especially after all the time and effort I had put into their businesses and the fact that I'd remained loyal to them after having been previously approached with other offers. I felt guilty for trying to do something for myself, but on the plus side I had a huge sense of relief, because it gave me time to go and explore all the things I wanted to do but couldn't while I was there.

As I left the salon on my last day and walked down by the seafront of Torquay with the sun beating down on my back,

I came past a restaurant that my best friend Ash worked at. I had to stop and tell him. As I did, I felt a smirk on my face as I realised I had done it. I felt free from all that anxiety that had been hanging over me.

I decided to sit there and have a drink while watching the sun reflect off the water. I watched the crowds of people strolling up and down the promenade. I just sat by myself for a minute or two, feeling free. It felt good. It felt right.

Starting the salon, however, was probably the most stressful thing I had ever done up to this point in my life. I was 28 and I had no guarantee it was going to work. I really didn't want to let my parents down – that was, and always had been, the biggest thing for me. It even got to the point where I developed a bit of a twitch in my eyelid from the stress of organising everything and trying not to forget anything for our opening day on 1st October 2011. I had a never-ending list and an ever-shrinking budget. I'm not going to lie; I felt the pressure. Even though I had quite a cool exterior, there was panic inside. A lot of it. Pretty much all the time.

I had never had to organise so much all at once. There was a lot more to do than I had bargained for. I hadn't even considered all the little bits and pieces I had to think about when opening a salon, all the things that are so important to the everyday, boring running of the ship. Just when I thought I'd got it all done, someone would say something and I'd think, *Oh no! We need an extra plug for that!* Or, *Oh shit! they haven't put the salon number on the door!* It seemed to go on forever.

Now, I could cut hair, but I had no idea about marketing, graphic design, interior design, health and safety, or all manner of other things! Time seemed to be running out fast.

We threw an opening party just a couple of days before we opened. I thought it would be good to have a date to work towards and also create a buzz before the shop opened its doors to the people of Torbay. It was a great idea, but it was another thing to add to my list. I had hoped that it would all be done and ready, with just a few things to finish off in the last few days.

The day arrived and there was a huge rush. My friend Ash helped out with food. We brought in bin liners full of ice and begged, stole, and borrowed everything we could. It was possibly the hottest September day ever, and the huge glass-fronted shop was heated up pretty well. It didn't help our ice efforts.

Most of the salon furniture hadn't arrived until that morning, and none of the mirrors were there for the event. I was devastated about this. *Oh my God! What are people gonna think?* I panicked. *A salon without mirrors!* But to my surprise no one mentioned it, and instead everyone just kept saying how great it was! (Thank God they arrived the next day, just in time for our 1st October opening day.)

It was amazing, really, that the party was such a huge success. It was great to see the place so busy that night, with all the team and all my family and friends filling up the salon – so much so that the party ended up spilling out onto the street! It was an incredible feeling, one that made me realise that I had done the right thing and that I had support for my decision. These guys had given up time to come and see our new venture. And on top of that, our new team had assembled together for the first time. That team – with a few changes along the way – would be at the core of the most important years of my career.

From then on, through lots of passion, time, and hard work, the salon grew in recognition and reputation. In fact, it turned into a massive success (if only from a personal viewpoint). It allowed me to have creative freedom, use the products I wanted, and to surround myself with the kind of genuine, passionate, and kind people I wanted in my team.

I also became an educator in the hair industry. This meant that I would share my knowledge, experience, and techniques learnt in classes. I wanted to share my secrets and give everyone who attended at least one new thing to take away from the class. It usually consisted of me giving two demos in front of experienced hairdressers, explaining the hows and whys of my methods. After lunch the learners would recreate the haircut on a live model. There are lots of different types of hair education – from "looks and learns" like that above, to platform work, which is a kind of show that normally lasts for a shorter period of time. There are also seminars about products, hair tools, and customer service or sales.

One of the main things that I loved doing – and that I now had that creative freedom to do – was photoshoots. The salon looked so impressive due to its industrial baroque interior that it always got a lot of attention. Often local photographers would come in, asking if they could take photos of the shop or use it for photoshoots. This happened a few times, until I met the fantastic Rob Grist at a wedding fair. He asked me if he could take some portraits of me, and from that moment on we developed a good friendship. We did lots of photoshoots together; some were on location, but more often than not we'd end up turning the salon into a studio. We'd come up with an idea or a theme, round up some models, and spend our Sunday creating a collection.

The first few collections we did were mostly for female hair, but for my 13-year anniversary in the hair industry I wanted to put together something a bit more special. Thirteen is my lucky number because it's the day I was born, plus I was just about to go into my second year of educating, so what better way to celebrate and promote this than with a collection of men's hair, and draw from it in my upcoming classes? I would use thirteen models from four different subcultures or tribes to showcase what I felt was current among my clientele.

With that idea in place, the project just grew and grew. The idea was to find models from the following groups: Rockabilly (or 50s inspired), Suited and Booted, Fitness, and finally Heavy Metal / Alternative. Luckily I had a very diverse group of mates and managed to find models for each of them. I then found out that a couple of them had old vintage cars that we could borrow for the shoot. One of the heavy metal guys had a Harley-Davidson, one of our fitness models ran a gym, and one of our suited and booted guys had a friend who was a tailor. It just all seemed to fall into place.

What if each section had its own location? I thought. And so I asked a local country mansion if we could come and shoot on site for the day. It was perfect. Half of Lupton House had been renovated and was very grand, with old wooden panelling and leather sofas surrounded by all the history. This really suited the smart, suited gents. And the parts of the house that *weren't* renovated were ideal for the heavy metal guys, with all the texture they offered: old plaster, exposed brick, and outbuildings with overgrown grass and plants. We then shot images of the rockabilly guys outside on the grounds; there was nothing modern in the background, so it could have been any time in history after the 1800s. It worked out great. For the fitness guys, we went early doors to the gym and shot a load of images in there of the guys working out both inside and outside of the gym.

However good these location shots were, both the photographer and I still felt that we needed at least one title studio shot, even if it was just one guy from each section. And so we brought the guys in again for one more day, recreating their looks and getting some images and video footage ready for the launch.

I was blown away by some of the images and I was very proud of the story we had built through this collection. Looking back now, I think we managed to capture the guys' identity really well, helping their personalities shine and letting them all show what it meant to be them.

Getting the photos back from any photographer always seems like a long wait – I was just dying to get them out there! But because I had taken a lot of images myself on my phone, I managed to put together some teaser videos using iMovie.

I made little short videos that were all well under a minute long and mixed them with some footage I got offline. I then started promoting the collection – which I named #th13teen – via social media, to try to raise some interest.

One day at the salon, I was cutting a client's hair and telling him about the shoot. I told him how much work had gone into it so far and I mentioned the launch.

'Why don't you use our bar for a launch party?' he asked me. 'We have a big screen you could use. We could do it on a Sunday night, so it won't disturb anything.'

Wow. A launch party for my collection? What a great idea, I thought to myself as I agreed wholeheartedly to the idea. And so we made it happen, not without a lot of stress – I had to put together the launch video with very basic video editing software that I'd taught myself to use, and it wasn't finalised until the next day. While planning the whole event, I always had that worry in the back of my mind. *Will people come?*

The atmosphere was great at the event, and the bar itself was perfect. Most of the models and their friends and family turned up and we had a live launch on the big screen, followed by a phenomenal performance by Seven Cities, my client's band.

It was absolutely priceless to have all of our hard work so well appreciated and to see the models' faces when their images went up on the big screen. The collection went on to be the first that I published in *Modern Barber* magazine, and I will never forget that. I will always be grateful to Rachel Gould, editor at the magazine, for that opportunity. It not only made me believe in myself and gave me confidence in my own work, but it also drove me to be featured again and again and to gain more coverage for my business.

This was my first big men's collection, and it set the bar for my forthcoming work. This experience cemented the idea that the best thing for me would be to move away from hairdressing – and that men's hair really was the way forward for my career.

CHAPTER 9

A LIFETIME OF DECISIONS

Opening Tom Chapman Hair Design was one of the best decisions I have ever made. It was also the place where I met Tenneille, my wife and mother of my two amazing sons.

I can still remember the day she walked in for her interview. I was completely blown away by her. It was probably the hardest interview I'd ever been involved in – from both sides. I could barely concentrate, and to top it all off she was a great hairstylist with skills and ability that made her perfect for the team. We became very good friends almost instantly, and we spent a lot of time with each other before we had any kind of romantic relationship. Despite this, I knew she was the one I wanted to be with from the very moment I met her. So, if nothing else, the salon gave me the thing that has made me the happier than anything else; the one thing that most of us desire – love.

Tenneille and I felt so connected right away. We spent all day every day together, working and living alongside one another. Her passion and drive always encouraged me to strive for more. Her belief in me alone enabled me to do so many things that are way out of my comfort zone.

In 2014, I knew that I wanted to ask her to marry me, so I decided to book a trip to Disneyland Paris. We had been to

Disney World the previous year and she fell in love with the place as much as I had. I can even remember us both crying when we came home because we wanted to go back so much! And so I surprised her with this trip to Disneyland Paris; and there were more tears as she opened up the *Frozen* Blu ray to the holiday tickets falling out.

I proposed to Tenneille on her favourite ride, Big Thunder Mountain. Now, if you've been to any Disney park or know anything about them, you'll know that this is a rollercoaster. My plan was to do it on the first lift. I had my sweaty hand in my pocket, clenched tightly around the ring that I had carried around with me for what seemed like forever and a day. When the train hit the lift, the click-clacking noise of the rollercoaster was so loud that I thought she'd never hear me, so I put the ring back into my pocket. Then, as we reached just over halfway, the noise quietened down. *Shit, this is my chance*, I thought to myself. *I'd better get this ring on her finger before we go over the edge and I bloody lose it!* Wrestling the ring out of my pocket and turning to Tenneille in a state of panic, I asked her the question.

Well, I shouted it at her.

'WILL YOU MAKE MY DREAMS COME TRUE?' I screamed at her. She had no chance to reply as we went over the edge, so I shoved the ring on her finger. She cried all the way round! We still have the ride photo as a memory.

When we got off the rollercoaster, she was actually able to say yes, so we went straight back on for another ride. Since then we've been to Disney World or Disneyland Paris four times in total, including on our honeymoon. Disney is most definitely our happy place and it holds so many memories for us, including our eldest son's first haircut. We couldn't decide whether Tenneille or I should cut it as we were both hairstylists, so instead, when we found out that getting your hair cut at Disney World means you get a certificate and special embedded Mickey ears, we decided he should have it done there. The Mickey ears now fit him, two years later.

Useless fact for you: as I write this – on 18th November 2018 – it is actually Mickey Mouse's 90th birthday.

Speaking of children, it was early in 2015 when we found out that my wife was pregnant. We didn't plan it, and originally it wasn't part of our plan at all. I wasn't sure it was the right thing for us, but I can remember seeing one of my clients come in with his two wonderful kids, and my heart melted. I realised I wanted that.

And so that was it. A few months later our son Abel was born; my Wonder Woman of a wife gave birth to our baby naturally, with no painkillers and without a single scream. She is a superhero!

CHAPTER 10

PAUSE FOR THOUGHT: PARENTHOOD

They say becoming a parent will change you forever, and they are right. Nothing can prepare you for that love and connection you have with that tiny person. You are introduced to a whole new world, a world of pride, love, fear, and a whole new concoction of emotions I never thought possible – being brought to tears of pride by the simplest of things, for one.

The love and connection between me and my child have grown, especially over the last 12 months. I will be honest and admit that at first it was love, no doubt, but there was not the connection I saw between mother and baby. I had an urge and want for that bond that seems so special, especially as my wife was breastfeeding. I sometimes felt a little on the outside, through no fault of anyone else. However, as my son has grown, so has the bond, and, talking to other men, I found that I was not alone in feeling this way. The time with him is so important, and I know that in this busy, consumerist lifestyle we lead, it is easy to be distracted by work and even buy him everything he wants – or what I think he wants – and needs.

As the bond has grown and he is now capable of showing his love in return, I am incredibly conscious that what he really desires are my time and attention. I look back to what an amazing childhood I had. When times were hard, we had some of the best fun because my parents spent a lot of time being creative and spending time with us doing some amazing things. When times were good, I was lucky enough to be part of their businesses, whether that was helping wait tables in their restaurant, or being an extra in a film and attending a night shoot with my dad when he had his film transport company.

This has made me realise that my best memories of my childhood are of times spent, not things owned.

No one says, 'I wish I'd spent less time with my family and worked more' on their death bed.

CHAPTER 11

RIP ALEX

One day in 2014, I had a conversation with my friend Alex. It went a little something like this.

'Hey! How's it going?' I asked.

'Not so bad, thanks,' Alex replied.

'Did you have a good time away?'

'Yeah, it was really good.'

'I've got to get back to work, buddy. My lunch break is over.'

'Yeah man, no worries!'

'See you.'

'Later, mate.'

Now, I'm not saying that this was our exact conversation – I'm sure there would have been some reference to wrestling in there. But it didn't consist of much more than that.

'Well, it was nice to see Alex – I'm so glad he had a good time away,' I said to my workmate, as we made our way back through Torquay town back to my salon, Tom Chapman Hair Designs.

I had no idea that it was going to be the last time I would see Alex before he took his own life.

A few nights later I jolted awake. I had just been drifting off when I noticed a lot of activity on my phone. Normally I would read on my phone in bed to try to clear my mind of the day's goings on, but I hadn't noticed anything odd. Now, though, Facebook notifications were flying in rapidly. I had to check out of curiosity, but when I saw what was causing all the activity, my heart sank.

There it was. "RIP Alex."

It rushed over me – that feeling of uncertainty and panic, where your chest feels like it's going to implode. I broke out in a cold sweat.

I saw the same comment again, from someone else.

"RIP Alex."

And again.

"RIP Alex."

And again.

"RIP Alex."

I didn't want to believe anything just yet. I frantically searched for a sign, some confirmation that Alex was alive. I wanted to know that this was all a mistake, or a rumour that had got out of control on social media. But the only confirmation I found was that he was no longer with us.

He had ended his own life. It was suicide.

I felt empty. I didn't want to believe it. Someone so young, someone so close to home, and someone so *fun* couldn't be gone! My heart raced and adrenaline rushed through my body; it was similar to that feeling when you have a heated confrontation when you're young.

The news was spreading like the plague; it travelled like wildfire among all of our friends online. The response was devastating.

Questions began hurtling through my mind as I sat up in bed.

If I had known that he was struggling, would I have paid more attention? Would I have given him more time?

Should I have been more aware, so that I could have realised what was going on?

Should I have given him more time to talk to me?

Could I have made a difference?

Why did he end his life?

What was he thinking when I saw him?

What was he thinking as he jumped?

With slightly awkward and sweaty digits, I tried to message those I knew from our teenage friendship group. I got hold of a couple of people who were obviously in as much shock as I was. They were clearly upset, judging by the typos in their rushed, erratic writing, full of grief and worry.

"He hasn't been happy for ages."

"I heard it was because of love life."

"Why didn't he say anything?"

"I think he was lonely."

"We should of done something, his poor family."

"I think it happened yesterday."

"I have no idea why heed do this he was fine the other day?"

No one I spoke to seemed to know what had happened, especially because, like in many of these situations, (especially online, where news can travel fast) there is a tendency for misinformation. Unfortunately, I don't think any of us will ever know why he did it. I just wish he hadn't. He was the first of our age group to go, and it was way too early.

I was in shock and feeling a certain level of guilt, as I had only seen him days before. I hadn't done anything for him – I hadn't even realised that there was anything wrong. We'd spent time together in the past and shared a love of wrestling, but despite our friendship, I still couldn't see what he was going through.

Why couldn't he tell me he was struggling? I don't necessarily mean that he should have told me something in that brief meeting during a lunch break, but why not before that? Why couldn't we have talked about this via an online message, text, or phone call? Why couldn't he speak to *anyone*?

Or maybe he did try to speak to his friends or family. Maybe he did try, but we all missed the cries for help.

I couldn't stay in bed any longer; I had to get up. I went to the lounge and sat there alone in silence for a while. At first, my mind felt blank. *Just be still for a while*, I thought. But then my senses were hit with an onslaught of information, as if the news had just hit me, hard. It felt as though I was flying at high speed, through a tunnel of blurred memories, emotions, thoughts, and feelings.

I continued to sit there in the dark, trying to find answers within my own mind.

Surprisingly I sniggered a bit to myself, remembering old times with him. I remembered all the times we debated who was the best hardcore wrestler or what was the greatest match of all time. Alex definitely had an opinion on things, and that included wrestling and music.

One particular event stood out in my memory. There was an altercation one night when we were out drinking. I can't remember what it was about, but as we were drunk and young, it was probably over a girl. I heard that Alex was out in the back of The Townhouse bar that we used to go to. Apparently, he was squaring up to another guy, who had plenty of back-up with him.

I went rushing down the slippery metal stairs as fast as my skintight drainpipe jeans would allow me, and split the whole thing up. Alex was much more slender than I was, so I easily picked him up and took him away from the action to cool off. As we sat there on the kerb around the corner, I managed to calm him down.

'What was that all about?' I asked.

Alex looked at me with a confused expression on his face and replied, 'I don't really know ...'

There were a few seconds of silence, and then we both just started laughing.

'You even don't know what was going on?' I asked him, chuckling. 'There were about five of them back there.'

'No,' he laughed back, shaking his head. 'I don't. Thanks for stopping it, though.'

I never did find out what had angered him so much. It's amazing what can happen when you're young and fuelled by testosterone and cider.

It was nice to remember times like these, but with the fond memories came the sudden realisation that this was it. This would be all that I would have of Alex from now on: just memories.

Now, I know that time had passed and we were both grown-up – I was spending all my time on my own business, and I had a fiancée – but even though we hadn't spent that much time together recently, it just felt so unfinished, so *final*.

A night of very little sleep and a lot of deep thought passed me by. In the morning I spoke to some more of our mutual friends on Facebook Messenger, hoping to get some kind of answer, or at least just some virtual company. Eventually I got up out of bed, showered, and went to work.

Maybe this was the wrong thing to do, I thought. *Maybe I should have taken some time out.* But I was always taught – both throughout my upbringing and by other, external influences in my life – that you're better to keep on working and keep yourself busy in times of loss or upset. 'It'll keep your mind off it all. Keep you active.' I suppose it does seem better than sitting there and wallowing in negativity, but personally I'm not sure it's a good thing to avoid negative emotions like this. In fact, I'm pretty sure it's not.

I am incredibly lucky, though, because although I have been almost hard-wired to "get on with things", I have a job where I spend a majority of my time talking and listening to my clients. I definitely believe that interaction helped me. I had all those people on whom I could offload my thoughts and feelings. I could speak to them about what I was experiencing. So although I was keeping busy, and although I wasn't resting up or taking time off – which admittedly *could* have benefitted me – I was in a place where I could talk to plenty of people and share the burden. I had the opportunity to get others' opinions instead of having these thoughts going round and round in my mind. It is astounding how much clarity you can get by sharing your thoughts.

I read recently that the average hairdresser / barber spends around 2,000 hours a year listening to people[i]. And I'm pretty sure most of them do the same amount of talking! The relationship you have with the person in your chair is pretty unique. There aren't many other careers like it. Your clients are, in a way, your friends, yet often not in your social circle. You are allowed into their personal space and they allow you a level of intimacy often only reserved for family or lovers. There is a level of unspoken confidentiality, because they know that what you talk about will never leave the shop. They trust you not only to come at them with sharp objects, but to style the hair that they'll be walking around with every day until their next visit.

Let's get that into perspective: you can change your clothes and your accessories – and even shave a beard off in your bathroom – on a daily basis, but your hair is the one constant stylistic thing that you take with you everywhere, every day. It is one of the first things people notice when they meet you. It's quite a big deal! So, as you might imagine, the relationship that is built between a hairstylist and their client is a strong one.

On that sad day I needed that closeness, that confidentiality. And so I spoke about Alex's death to each and every one of my clients. On an average day I can style up to 12 clients, most of whom I have known for many years and have a strong relationship with. This means that on that day, I spoke to around 12 people about Alex, about his death, about the fact that I had spoken to him days earlier and not noticed that anything was wrong. I told them about the guilt I felt, wondering how bad things must have been for him to feel that he had to take his own life.

I'm not saying that I *vented* to everyone, or poured my whole heart out. But they asked me how I was, as I did with them. I learnt that other people had experienced this. Other people had lost friends and family to suicide; other people had thought about taking their own life. Some offered me support, should I have needed it.

I'm in a very privileged position. I know I have a support circle, but speaking to my clients and hearing it from them was something different altogether. I knew it went both ways too, as I had spent the day listening to their stories and experiences as well. It was like a series of small, intimate, one-off support groups where we could offload, enabling each of us to move on a little each time.

Going to work that day was the best thing I could have done. I fear that having the day off by myself, alone with all those questions and thoughts going around in my head, would have been far worse. Instead I spoke to people and I didn't avoid what I was thinking or feeling.

At the end of that day, I felt a little less lost and empty.

CHAPTER 12

THE FUNERAL

When the day of the funeral actually came, it all still felt like a bad dream – and a hazy one at that. But it did feel final.

I had actually worked on the morning of that day; I'd been behind the chair cutting hair as usual. It's kind of my safe place, a time where all I have to think about is my client in the chair and about our conversation. That morning we did talk about the impending funeral, but it was nice to be there discussing it instead of at home worrying about it.

I finished my last client and got changed. The problem was that I didn't actually own a plain black shirt at the time and the closest thing I had was a black Hawaiian shirt. It was mostly black, but it also had green and pink flowers on it. I was incredibly self-conscious about this. *I can't turn up like this*, I fretted. But I'd had no time to get to a shop beforehand.

In my worry, I messaged a few of our friends who were also going to the funeral. 'What do you think?' I asked them. 'I don't think Alex would care, but what about the family?'

Thankfully, they all replied and told me that they didn't think Alex or the family would care at all. In fact, Alex would probably approve as it was more punk rock! And so with that in mind, I made my way to the crematorium in Torquay. It was the first funeral I had attended since I lost my grandad.

As I turned the corner and walked towards the crematorium, I saw the sheer number of people who were all waiting to go inside. I was blown away. *All these people are here for him, but he still had to suffer alone?* I thought to myself as I sheepishly joined the flock.

Although I now make a living from going on stage and speaking in front of people, I used to be very insular at times, and I still am in certain situations. Often, I find it difficult time to know what to say or how to start a conversation – especially when you're among a bunch of young people in their twenties, all waiting to say goodbye to a friend who took his own life, all feeling a little helpless and lost. We hadn't all been together in one place for many years. There was a lot of hugging, crying, and questioning. In fact, one question in particular kept arising: 'Why does it take something like this for us all to get together again?'

We all told each other that we'd make more of an effort, but of course there probably hasn't been another get-together since. If there has been, I know I wasn't there.

Unfortunately, life and its commitments get in the way. When you're younger and living at home there are no responsibilities and life is far freer and simpler, even if you don't feel that at the time.

The time had come to enter the crematorium and say farewell to Alex. As we filed in and more and more people were ushered into the room, it became apparent how many mourners were actually there. We realised that there just wasn't going to be enough room for everyone; all the seats were full and the crowd were being directed towards the front.

'Oh no, I don't wanna be stood up down the front,' I said, starting to panic at the pressure of being next to Alex in front of everyone. 'I can't be.'

But I had no choice. I ended up being wedged in right next to his coffin. It was boiling in there with all those people inside and

I still had my coat on. I didn't want to disturb anyone by taking it off in such a small space. With the heat, the worry that I hadn't taken my coat off, the strangeness of being so close to Alex and the emotion of the occasion, I was sweaty and flustered to say the least.

The service itself was excellent and the priest (or vicar – I'm not sure which he was) was on great form. It probably wasn't his usual audience or his normal choice of music, considering that Alex had been into punk rock. I'm pretty sure Alkaline Trio hadn't been played in Torquay Crematorium before then – and maybe even since!

Although it was a great send-off, it was truly devastating. From where I was sitting, I could see the heartbreak that surrounded me on all sides. It was a strange perspective, being at the front and looking back at everyone else. Everywhere I looked I saw tears, red faces, heads in hands, and blank expressions. I could feel the anger and sadness that radiated from everyone. Paradoxically, emptiness filled the room.

I scanned the room, making eye contact with our closest friends. Every so often I would get a nod of recognition, which felt like a comforting arm around my shoulder. It was as if they all wanted to say, 'I know, mate. It's shit, ain't it?' I received mostly blank stares from behind a veil of tears from almost everyone else.

My memory from this point is a bit hazy at best. We all got through the service and filed out of the room, saying our final goodbyes to Alex. We took only our memories with us, ready to be shared openly at the wake.

From what little experience I have of funerals, it seems that the atmosphere changes an awful lot from the funeral to wake. I'm not sure why, and I'm certain that others might see this in a different light, but at the wake it almost feels like a load has been lifted. Those in attendance start to focus on the best things about the ones they have lost. And this occasion was no different.

We all arrived at the local pub, which had a function room out the back, and we all piled in. It was exactly what I had imagined a British pub party to be – there was a buffet of British classics, such as Scotch eggs and mini pasties, laid out on a long table along with paper plates. There was also a dance floor that wouldn't get used until most people were far too drunk to walk, let alone dance.

We gathered together into our closer friendship groups, and that's when things became a little more light-hearted. We reminisced about past nights out and live music gigs. We shared our grief and stressed how much Alex would be missed.

How could this have happened to him, without any of these people knowing about it? I thought to myself. *I need to do something*.

'I need to do something for Alex,' I said out loud to the group. 'Something needs to be done to remember him. Maybe I can organise an event in his memory or something, to raise awareness about this tragedy.'

'You'll do something, we know you will,' one friend said to me.

Another added, 'You're good at organising things and getting people together. Let us know and we'll be there.'

I couldn't have imagined at that point where I would be 12 months later, and what I would go on to create for myself and many others.

CHAPTER 13

THE LION'S PRIDE

It was late August 2015; I had been educating in men's hair for about a year, and I was starting to delve deeper into the subculture of barbering. It was growing into a movement. It was new and exciting, and it felt like a whole new community. I'd started looking online for tips, information, and ways of improving my classes so that I could give more to those who attended.

Among this online community I found a Facebook group called New World Barbers. There were some phenomenal barbers in the group, and I was inspired just by looking at the standard of work on there. This gave me an idea: what if I could get all these guys to donate an image of a haircut they had done and create a lookbook? Not only would customers be able to choose a new style from the collection of pictures, but the book would showcase some great barbers to boot. Plus, I could hopefully sell it and raise money for charity at the same time!

So, after some consideration, I posted in the group looking for barbers who were interested in being part of the collection. To my knowledge, nothing like this had ever been done before, and I wasn't sure if anyone would be interested. However, the response I got was unbelievable – there was so much interest from so many top barbers! I almost couldn't believe that some of these guys were talking to me, let alone considering my idea. It made me feel included in that community.

We gathered a pride of 30 multi-award-winning, widely published, well-established and experienced barbers from all over the UK and Ireland, and even one from the Netherlands. I invited them all into an online group chat. I was a little nervous that I was supposed to "lead" this group – in my mind, I was the least experienced, least qualified and least well known among them all. But I was lucky to have some guidance from a guy from Ireland who had been dubbed "The Godfather of Irish Barbering" in the most recent issue of *Barber NV* magazine. His name was Pat, and he was well known in the industry and had a lot of experience. He was excited by the project and wanted to be on board; at the start he and I spent a lot of time on the phone running through ideas. Pat kept telling me how big this all could be, and he gave me a lot of advice.

Much to my surprise, I now had a group of barbers to work on the lookbook. It was actually happening. Now we just needed a name and a charity to work with. I threw these both out for discussion in the group. There was an onslaught of suggestions when it came to charities, but it was a little quiet on the name front – although the word "collective" came up a lot. Then one barber – Paul Mac of Ireland – came up with a great suggestion. It hit me so hard I couldn't believe I hadn't thought of it.

"'The Lions". Just like the rugby team. What do you think?' he asked. It made perfect sense – barbers from all over the UK and Ireland had come together to form a team, just like the British Lions.

And so it was agreed, and at that moment The Lions Barber Collective was born.

I didn't realise at that point that the name would be so strong and go on to have so many other meanings. It fit so well into what we were doing – creating a pride. We would later develop something called the Lions Dens drop-in groups, and have associations with courage and bravery in so many stories and within so many cultures. It was just *right*, and continues to be so today.

Being barbers, we agreed on the idea that we would raise money for a men's charity, but the ideas coming from the group all seemed to be around men's cancer. To be fair, this was a very worthy cause, but I felt there was so much already out there for cancer. I wanted something that was not only fresh, but which needed that awareness or funding.

And then Paul came up with a second great suggestion. Why didn't we support a suicide prevention charity?

What a fantastic idea! It had only been about a year since I had personally lost a friend to suicide – how had suicide prevention not occurred to me before? Well, perhaps I do know the reason – it was partly because I was completely unaware of any services that existed, and partly because I didn't know it was even a thing to be a suicide prevention service in the first place. I hadn't even really considered mental health at all, but it seemed so obvious now.

My mind was made up. If I had been affected by losing a friend to suicide and was completely unaware of these services and organisations that existed, how many others were out there in the same boat? How many were suffering in silence, or even actively searching for help but unaware of the services available? I just really wanted to raise awareness about what people could do for support. What charities existed? Maybe we could potentially raise some money to help them?

I knew I wanted a smaller charity that would really benefit from whatever we could give them, and so I decided to go with Papyrus, a suicide charity for young people. I told Papyrus my ambition, and that we could potentially raise thousands of pounds for them. They were obviously thrilled.

We had the idea, we had the barbers, we had the name, and we had the cause. Now, we just needed to create the book. Easy, right?

Far from it. As it turned out, the journey I had set out on would be one of the hardest, most time-consuming and stressful ones I would ever undertake.

CHAPTER 14

DISASTER

We announced The Lions Barber Collective on 10th September 2015, on World Suicide Prevention Day.

It seemed like things were all just falling into place. That morning I had a telephone interview with the journalist Martin Daubney for a piece in *The Telegraph*; they'd contacted me and asked if I'd like to do a piece with them. I had no idea how these things were happening – people were just getting in contact with me! Still to this day I have never had to do a hard sell about our cause or method, and it's a good job as well, because I am *awful* at it.

People were standing up and paying attention, and they wanted to know more. It's pretty amazing, to be honest. People see our passion – and the fact this all genuinely means a lot to me – and it works.

Very quickly after the inception of The Lions, I had realised that not only could we raise awareness of men's mental health, but we also had such a great opportunity to actually help clients in a way that could potentially save lives.

It is often joked that barbers or hairstylists act as counsellors and therapists as well. And even though it's mostly meant as a joke, it is most definitely true. For some people in our chairs, the level of human connection and trust is so high that they feel comfortable enough to be able to speak freely to their barber or hairdresser. Often the relationship is long-term, with a return rate of every few weeks. And however often you see a client, it's rare that you know them outside the four walls of the shop. The bond is therefore strong, but there is a disconnection between you and your client's friendship group. This, combined with client confidentiality, means that there is little worry that what they share with you is going to make it back to their friends or family.

The barbershop is a safe environment, one that offers a kind of connection that we are experiencing less and less every day. There is physical and verbal communication, a certain unique level of trust (you have to make sure they look great when they leave your shop!) and no interruptions. This is why the barber chair is such an important and invaluable place to support mental health and suicide prevention.

On top of that, it's in a far less depressing environment than the places that some other support groups take place. And so we went on to create something called The Lions' Den in the salon; a drop-in support group which we held every last Friday of the month during opening hours, with a voluntary mental health professional on site. The idea was that the barbershop is a completely non-clinical environment in which you won't be judged, diagnosed or anything else. Plus, a barbershop waiting area is a normal place for guys to sit and chat anyway, so who has to know that you're attending a support group if you want the fact to remain unknown?

I felt the need to create some ways in which we could let other barbershops get on board. The message was that anyone could help those in their chairs by being a non-judgemental listener, but people really wanted to belong to the pride. That was an amazing feeling, but it meant that I had to come up with something concrete. Obviously as a charity we had to be careful, especially as we were dealing with a subject as sensitive and important as suicide and mental health. I also had to think about how I could protect the wellbeing of the Lions themselves, as well as the clients who spoke to them.

There seemed to be a lot to think about, but I thought a good place to start would be to invite other barbershops to start doing some of the things that we did locally already. What if we made The Lions' Den a national thing, and have people sign an agreement to protect all those involved?

In order to sign up to this initiative and join The Lions Barber Collective, all you needed to do was find a volunteer mental health worker to give you their time and set up a Lions' den. And that is it. It was effectively a simple idea which allowed others to get on board initially without having to do much except open their doors to their community. We gained plenty of interest, and still we are always looking for more barbers to offer a Lions' Den at their location.

I was in awe of the number of guys who became part of The Lions Barber Collective, and now I was up in the early hours of the morning on the phone to *The Telegraph* – in my pants nonetheless – to announce the creation of this new barber movement, one that was supporting men's mental wellbeing. It was surreal to say the least, and it was to become a whirlwind of a journey over the next couple of years.

I was starting to feel the pressure. It was real now. The world knew about our new initiative and our plans for the lookbook – and now I'd have to follow through with it. I couldn't fail! The timing might not have been perfect (when is it ever?) as my wife was eight months pregnant, but I knew I had to get our lookbook created.

This task meant that I had to manage 30 barbers, getting them all to take a hi-res photo of a haircut they had done. To keep a level of synergy throughout the book and curate a "collection", I suggested that everyone donate a black-and-white image with their model wearing a black T-shirt. A friend then suggested that each barber should find themselves a sponsor for their page, in order to help us raise the money we needed for the design and print of the book. I thought it was a fantastic idea. It would mean the book would be self-funded, and anything raised from it would be able to go to Papyrus.

I myself had created a lot of photoshoots and collections by that point, so I naturally assumed that it was fairly simple to get a hi-res image in black and white. But you should never assume! A lot of the guys had never done a photoshoot before and were unaware of how hi-res imagery worked, and so I was sent a lot of photos that just weren't high quality enough. Some of the guys just sent iPhone pictures. This meant that, although the haircuts were phenomenal, the quality of the images was nowhere near good enough for print. This resulted in a lot of back and forth and, as you can imagine, that took a long time. It caused me plenty of stress.

But this was the first time I had organised such a thing. The concept was new to a lot of people involved, and so naturally mistakes get made in such situations. We had originally set a deadline of 31st October 2015, but we had nowhere near all the images we needed when that day arrived. These men were all top barbers by trade, so they led extremely busy lives themselves, and finding the time to set aside a day for a professional shoot instead was incredibly difficult. As a result, we kept having to extend the deadline so that we could get enough content to make the book worthwhile. We really needed it to look like a real collection.

To top this all off, my son was born on the 22nd October 2015, so I wasn't getting much sleep! Thank God my wife was incredible and supported everything I was doing.

The sponsor idea was also proving difficult – we were completely new and we had a new idea, and although we'd had a phenomenal reaction to the inception of The Lions Barber

Collective, we were definitely not established or proven. We did manage to get some support though, including sponsorships from Keune, Andis, and Millennium. There *was* some support out there for us.

The project dragged on and on, and month after month went by. With Christmas on the horizon, there was little chance of it getting done by the end of the year. I was highly conscious of this when I was pestering the guys, asking them when their photos would be available. I must have spent hundreds of hours on Facebook Messenger alone! My focus was to get this project done, dusted, and out there – even if (ironically) it was probably not great for my mental health.

There was a constant worry at the back of my mind. It often popped up as soon as my head hit the pillow at night. My biggest worry was letting people down and not delivering what I'd said I would. There was also the added pressure of this book being made for charity. I had been incredibly hyped up about the whole thing, and my friend Pat had had such a bright vision of it all. Instead, the reality right now was nothing but stress and worry.

Sometimes I wished I'd never started it.

When I finally had all the images, I had to enlist the help of a designer in order to put them together. I had no idea how I was going to do it, but thankfully Paul Mac came to rescue once more. Paul put me in touch with a guy he knew who ran a magazine in Ireland, and what's more, he was willing to do the work for me for free because it was for charity! What a huge relief!

Paul's friend was brilliant and put the full book together for us. Since I was a complete amateur, he was patient with the process, and spent quite a lot of time on the phone with me after we had sent all the images, names, sponsors, and other information over to him. Paul also shot the front cover for the book.

I myself had taken a quick shot at my own photoshoot as an afterthought. I wanted to show someone whispering into a barber's ear and wearing a Lions T-shirt; the idea being that our clients can speak to us openly without fear of judgement. Paul really liked the idea and decided to recreate the image – and he absolutely smashed it. It really made the project and I was so pleased with the outcome. When I saw the developing layout, I started to feel like it was nearly over. Soon I could get back to some kind of normality.

When I was sent the final PDF of the lookbook, it seemed like such a huge landmark. I'd been promising this thing to the world for months, and now it was finally here and ready to be printed. What a relief! I had made it! All that hard work and organising was done and dusted.

This wasn't the end of the project, though, not by a long shot. Luckily – with help from Andrew Brewster, who was in charge of *Barber NV* magazine at the time – we got the pennies together to get the book printed (apparently it costs a lot more than I expected) and managed to send the PDF off to the printers. Andrew fronted some of the money for me so that I could get them printed and pay the difference back after the launch, with the rest of the money going to the charity.

At this point the biggest barber-only industry show, Barber Connect, was fast approaching. This was our big chance to get it out there for the masses of barbers in attendance. I had been approached by the great guys at BarberBlades (an industry wholesaler who organises the event) and asked if we would be interested in having a stand at the expo, which was to take place at the prestigious Celtic Manor Hotel in Wales.

This was mind-blowing to me. I had always suffered with a bit of imposter syndrome in the barbering world. I worried that I'd get "found out", that they'd realise I was a hairdresser by trade and that my barber skills were self-taught. I didn't do shaving and I believed that I wouldn't be taken seriously if they knew. I was still only a learner barber, and at that point I didn't see the benefits of being a hairdresser. I couldn't see that my current

BarberTalk | **Tom Chapman**

skills were helping me to progress. And so having this invitation felt welcoming, as though I'd been accepted into the barbering world. We all want to belong, and I was incredibly lucky to be welcomed into the barbering world with open arms.

There was only one problem: it was the same weekend as my wedding.

Now, at first there was talk of me leaving the day after the wedding and heading up to the show, in order to ensure that everything went well. However unrealistic this was, I felt I'd need to know that it was all going smoothly to put my mind at rest. However, after much discussion and assurance from a friend (a fellow Lion and a driving force behind the lookbook) that it would all go to plan, I decided that I wouldn't go. It was my wedding, after all, and I really wanted to be with my new wife and enjoy the day to its fullest with no distractions.

The weekend came, starting with the evening of the wedding on the Saturday. We got married in our back garden, so there was a lot of work to do. I had had my son overnight and the groomsmen had all stayed at my house, so I decided that it was best for me to stay away from social media. I needed to concentrate on the wedding, not the Barber Connect event, even if it was the launch of the long-awaited lookbook. There were way more important things to concentrate on.

To add to it all, my eight-month-old son was ill and basically slept on me all night. It was lovely, but it meant little to no sleep for me.

The next morning came and we got everything in order with plenty of time. I'm not going to lie, I was a bit worried about Barber Connect, but I was reassured it would all be fine. I decided to resist the urge to go online and just enjoy the day after all. I had sent all the banners, stickers, leaflets, and other materials to the venue, and had received confirmation that the lookbook would be delivered to our stand at the event ready for the weekend.

The wedding was beautiful – the best day ever – even though I'd had very little sleep. And that was on top of the worrying thoughts going through my mind: *Will the wedding run smoothly? Will the launch of the book go well?*

All in all, we had a beautiful day with our families and spent the whole day and night celebrating. To top it off, I hadn't heard anything from Barber Connect, so I assumed all was well and everything had arrived and was in place. The event wasn't until the Sunday and Monday, and the last thing I saw was that some of the Lions guys had checked in at Celtic Manor. Others were on their way there.

No news is good news. Or so I thought.

The day after our wedding, my new wife and I returned to the house after a lovely breakfast spent looking out to sea at the hotel that Tenneille's dad kindly surprised us with. We then spent a day at home together, reflecting on the excellent day before. Thankfully we had hired a cleaner and therefore the carnage we had left was basically all sorted on our return that Sunday morning.

Later that night, after a long relaxing day, I thought to myself, *I'll check Facebook and see how everything's going*. I couldn't resist it any longer – I needed to know. The Sunday was the first day of the two-day event which had thousands of attendees. I'd had hundreds of Lions logo stickers printed, with the idea that all those passing the stand could put them on their shirts. That way we would have a huge presence on all the social media photos, whether we were tagged or not. Our logo would be everywhere.

But there was nothing online. *Odd*, I thought. *But hey, maybe they forgot them, or people didn't want to cover themselves in stickers?* Fair enough.

Then I turned my notifications back on. And my heart stopped.

A flood of messages came through, and I feared the worst immediately. I didn't want to read them; I just wanted to go on and enjoy my time with my wife. But I couldn't ignore it. I needed to know. So I bit the bullet and delved into my messenger inbox.

There were lots of stories coming through with slight variations, but all to the same end: the Lions' stand – the one that had been donated to us in an amazing location, with the value of well over £1,000 – had been unmanned all day. Empty. No one had been there.

The organisers were understandably furious. The other original Lions – those who were in attendance and had planned to demonstrate haircuts on the stand – had had nowhere to cut because there were no chairs there. There was also no one there to direct things. The person who had assured me everything would be okay was nowhere to be found.

My heart sank. What a kick in the balls! In a few minutes I'd gone from being on a high from the wedding and spending a wonderful day with my new wife, to feeling alone and let down. It was a complete disaster.

To top all of this off, the box of lookbooks had been delivered to the empty stand – where someone had opened them. They'd nearly all been taken because people had just assumed that they were free!

We were screwed.

We needed to make the money to pay off the rest of the printing costs, which Andrew had kindly paid for us in advance, and now we had no chance of doing it. I had just paid for a wedding, and it was looking like we would have to use our wedding money to pay for these lost books. I was devastated to say the least. How the fuck was I going to tell my new wife?!

At that point, I nearly gave it all up. *Could it all really be worth this?* I asked myself. The idea was to help those struggling with their mental health, not completely destroy mine! I felt broken and completely let down. I even felt like a bit of a fool.

As I started to delve into the messages and speak to others, I got so many replies. Each of them tried to explain what had happened or how people had tried to help out throughout the day.

If it wasn't for those messages of support from some brilliant barbers who I look up to, I don't know what I would have done. That really made me realise that I wasn't alone. I was shown such kindness by the guys from Reuzel, a hair product brand. They had been cutting hair on their stand and raising money all day, which they then donated to us. It was a huge surprise and also took the edge off a little. Then there were the efforts of Jac Ludlow, who saved the remaining books and found all the Lions banners and other materials for me, even though I was told that they'd never arrived.

It was such a huge relief. If we had lost them too, we would have been so out of pocket it would've been soul destroying. I will never be able to thank Jac enough for that day. He restored my faith and went out of his way to make things better for me. Without that I don't know what I would have done. All I know is that I would have been completely defeated.

I was utterly broken when I thought about all the hours I had put into what we were doing. I couldn't believe that this had happened! *How* could it have happened?

Rightly or wrongly, I decided to do some digging to try to find out what had gone wrong. I was horrified that the stand had been empty all day, and I couldn't find or contact the guy who was supposed to have been in charge of it. I kept calling him but I got no answer at all. His last-known whereabouts were apparently in the bar the previous night, so I knew he had made it to the venue, but he hadn't been seen since. To say I was disappointed was an understatement. I felt ashamed and embarrassed.

This guy that I had looked up to and admired had completely abandoned us all on this huge landmark in the calendar of The

Lions Barber Collective. I had no idea what to do except panic. *What will people think of me and the Lions?* I fretted. *How would we ever come back from this? Would I ever be respected in the industry? There's surely no way we would ever be able to attend any more industry events again after this almighty cock-up!*

Luckily, I managed to get hold of the organisers and apologise. They were incredibly understanding due to the wedding, considering their financial loss. I'm sure they felt pretty stupid as well, having donated a stand to a group that were a complete no-show.

My wife was unbelievable. She has supported me through so much since we found each other, but she really made all the difference on that day. She calmed me down, encouraging me to speak to people online and find out what had happened. She talked me out of quitting and closing down The Lions Barber Collective altogether. She convinced me that we would see it through and come out the other side. It made me realise that I was lucky to have her.

Eventually we figured out that the Lion left in charge had grasped the entirety of his actions and had decided to hide in his room. And although I'll never know the real truth, I was hearing many, many stories about his antics the night before the event. By the next day I still hadn't had any messages from him. Not a sausage. I was fuming.

Then, on Monday evening, I heard from another Lion who had been there as well. He informed me that the guy who had let me down had been ill, and was in fact calling a doctor to his room to try to get him medically cleared to fly. I was sceptical to say the least, especially after hearing stories about him being in the bar and watching the football, but still I felt I needed to give him the benefit of the doubt, even though he hadn't contacted me himself.

Now, I totally understand if someone is ill and cannot attend a planned event. But I was upset that he didn't think to contact any one of the twenty or so Lions at the expo and let them know that he couldn't make it. Couldn't they possibly have grouped together and manned the stand throughout the day, get the banners and other material, and decorate it all? There must have been a way! They had even told people that they couldn't dress the stand because I hadn't sent the stuff over. That hurt me. I had spent so much time on this event, alongside organising a wedding and having my first child. I had given it my everything.

Once the event was over, I finally got the chance to speak to the Lion in question on the phone. I accepted his apology, but I let him know how I felt after all the energy I had put into everything since the inception. It felt like he was riding the coattails of it all.

To be totally honest, there wasn't much more to the conversation. I hate confrontation and try to avoid it as much as possible. I squirm at the very thought of it. I just told him how upset I was. He didn't come back with much either, other than accepting what I said.

It did make me reassess our relationship and his role within The Lions Barber Collective, but a few weeks later we were due to fly to Chicago for the B-Groomed grooming event. This was a first-time event for male grooming in the USA, and this same guy who had messed up at Barber Connect had organised for The Lions Barber Collective to attend B-Groomed and have a stand. The guys who organised the event kindly paid for our travel and hotel and printed off some banners and backdrops for us. They were really good to us and provided a platform for us to meet so many others in the industry.

As well as promoting our charity work, my fellow Lion and I would be presenting a class together and doing a presentation on stage. I certainly wasn't going to miss out on the opportunity to raise awareness and make new connections, but I was aware of the bad vibe between us and was worried about confrontation, despite the fact that I wanted to speak to him about it in person. Because of this – and since it would be the first time I had seen him in person since the incident – I felt I should wait until then and see how things went. I was dreading seeing him when I arrived.

Things didn't improve on that trip. I realised that he could no longer be part of what I was trying to do if we were to take things further. I had worked hard on putting a presentation together for the class and organising a lot for our piece on stage, but in return he put in little effort. His attitude towards the Lions wasn't what I needed if I was going to make it a success. He had influenced a lot of the decisions and had some great ideas, but now I really wanted to do everything for the right reasons with the right people.

It was time to start afresh and try to take it to the next level by myself. The lookbook project had been utter chaos, but I realised it was the start of something much bigger. We had started to build a platform from which I could push forward and grow the Lions into something special.

One amazing thing did happen on that trip to Chicago: I met a man called Lawrence Fo and I instantly hit it off with him. When you spend the week in a small room at the Freehand Hotel – just four barbers in bunk beds, with one bathroom and no storage – you really get to know one another. He helped no end all week; he manned the stand with me, helped with the class we took, and helped me do some interviews. He was even there to support me through the pressure and worry of dealing with the Lion that had let me down.

We laughed a lot, shared stories, and had a few adventures while there, such as joining a Black Lives Matter walk when we had just planned to step outside while he smoked a cigarette. People kept asking if we were in a band, so after a while we just went with it, telling them we were a band called Snail Trail and that it was our first tour of the USA. There's no doubting that Chicago is now one of my favourite cities, partly because of the fun that I had with Lawrence.

Lawrence himself had been misdiagnosed for years before finally receiving the correct bipolar diagnosis. His story fascinated me, especially the part where he'd come off the medication that had turned him into the uncreative, overweight zombie and instead became the inspirational global educator and platform artist he is now. The drugs had stopped his mania but had also stopped him from doing anything at all really. He had no drive left; he was just existing. He gave me a great insight into his amazing life, his ongoing recovery, and coping mechanisms. The fact that he had made such a success of himself and used his bipolar disorder to his advantage was so inspiring.

It really was a fantastic insight into how sometimes medication and diagnosis may not be the best route for everyone. It was hard to imagine him as overweight and "zombie-like"; he just had so much life and creativity in him. He was so passionate about what we were trying to do with the Lions that he became an integral part of the next phase of the Collective as we turned the page and began a new chapter. In fact, Lawrence has become a great ambassador for The Lions. He has even been featured on Sky News, talking about his story and ours as well. I am so proud to know Lawrence and consider myself lucky to have met him. His strength, integrity, and kindness to those less fortunate is like no other.

The Chicago trip was a real eye-opener. I couldn't believe the interest we'd had from people in the UK, let alone the interest we had there in Chicago. We even ended up being invited down to FOX, thanks to the marketing and media guys for the B-Groomed event. They very kindly asked if we would be interested in joining them and discussing how we hoped to connect with men in the barber chair and use our unique position to save lives.

The next morning, I was up early and suited and booted. I whisked across Chicago to a huge building, where I found myself in the studio talking about the Lions live on the morning news.

I'd actually be lying if I said I was nervous this time – for once, that anxiety didn't hit me. I don't know why exactly, but all I can gather is that, because no one I knew would be watching, I didn't feel any pressure. Does that make sense? Being live on a TV show that's going out to millions of viewers is no pressure apparently!

As I sat in the green room waiting to go on, the reality of what I was doing hit me. I walked past all the framed pictures of FOX's hit shows, including *The Walking Dead* and *Family Guy*. Then, once we were all mic'd up, we entered the studio. It was like walking onto the set of *Anchorman*! The guys put us all at rest and gave us directions, and then the next thing I knew, I was sitting in front of the camera next to the presenters, reading the autocue and waiting for my turn to speak.

When the host turned to me, she asked me what was going on at the B-Groomed event.

'We've got a hell of a lot going on at the B-Groomed Men's Expo event,' I told her. 'We've got live music, we've got barbers, we've got barber battles, we've got DJ battles, we've got a beard contest with Fit for Vikings – he's a real Icelandic Viking. He makes his own beard care products, and he's going to do one with us for the Lions Barber Collective, to raise awareness for suicide prevention and men's mental health. There's going to be loads of stuff going on.'

'Let's talk about the foundation that all this stuff is benefitting to,' the host said. 'Because guys go to barbershops, and just like women do at beauty salons, they talk to their barber. And maybe they've got stuff heavy on their mind, and this is something that's near and dear to you guys.'

'Yeah, of course it is,' I replied. 'I founded the Lions Barber Collective last year, and Pat helped hugely with driving things forward. I lost a friend to suicide a couple of years ago. He had so many friends, but he didn't have anyone to talk to. So, this is where we've developed the idea for BarberTalk training, which is teaching barbers to be able to recognise the signs of depression, mental ill-health and the early signs of suicide, so that they are able to ask people direct questions, listen non-judgmentally, and then signpost them to all these amazing organisations that are out there. It's such a problem and men are scared to talk about their problems because they're perceived to be weak.'

'What an awesome outlook you guys are providing!' said the host.

It was a fantastic experience and it flew by – we were even invited to take part in the weather report! I felt such a rush as we left those studios, right in the heart of Chicago, and headed back over to the event.

After we came off I spoke to a couple of people at the studios who congratulated us on the idea of utilising the barbershop and the relationship between barbers and clients. While on the news we had limited time, but it was just enough for me to get a fair bit out about The Lions Barber Collective and the shocking statistic that someone takes their life every 12.3 minutes in the USA, which was correct at the time. I have just read on the American Foundation of Suicide Prevention website that the number is now 123 suicides a day at the time of writing.[ii]

Looking back, I think this positive experience at FOX was exactly what I needed after what had happened. It kind of closed one chapter and began another. It gave me clarity in myself and my mind, and I knew where I was going from there.

When I returned, I had to clean up the mess by paying for the books out of my own money. I then managed to get hold of the guys who ran BarberBlades and they agreed to sell the remainder of the lookbooks. Jac Ludlow so kindly delivered to them for me, and they sold out of the remaining few books through their barber equipment distribution company. We then donated the money that we raised to Papyrus. Once this was done, it felt like some kind of symbolism for closure.

The lookbook may have been the inaugural project of the Lions, but it had become poisonous and draining. But I know I am wiser because of my experiences, which at least means I have gained something from the whole affair. There have since been talks of doing another one, but I'm not keen. I might consider doing it at a later date, but most definitely in a completely different way.

Now I could finally draw a line under the whole thing and follow my passion and drive. I could try to make a difference in the future.

I wanted to do right by Alex's memory.

CHAPTER 15

PAUSE FOR THOUGHT: FAILURE

I spend most of my days behind the chair in conversation with many different people from all walks of life. Recently I was told about a child's birthday party, where a game of musical chairs took place. Only, they did not remove a single chair, ensuring that each child had a chair of their own every time the music stopped.

It made me wonder: why was this necessary? To avoid disappointment, breakdowns, or tantrums? When would the game end? Were there winners and losers? And are we so afraid of failure?

Contemplating this more, I recalled when I was training to become an assessor, and on that course the lecturer said, 'If the student doesn't pass, they ...'

Fail, I thought.

'... set up a scheduled learning plan for the next assessment,' she continued.

What is so wrong with failure, and why are we avoiding it with our children and students? Because as soon as we are adults, failure is commonplace in most walks of life, and it's not a bad thing.

Have you ever wondered why air travel is the safest form of transport? It all comes down to the black box. The black box records all the information between the plane and the air traffic control team, as well as the complete sound and dialogue of the cockpit. If there were any mistakes, accidents, or, God forbid, a crash, all that content is available to anybody from any nation to assess, research, and investigate – and they do every time. The crew are held accountable, and the blame is not shifted to others or avoided all together.

In fact, they see failure as the very best way to learn. Rather than denying their mistakes, blaming others, or attempting to spin their way out of trouble, these institutions and individuals interrogate errors as part of their future strategy for success, which has led to air travel being incredibly safe and improving all the time.

In 2015 there were 560 deaths in air travel. However, 374 of these were in deliberate crashes or bombs, meaning only 186 deaths globally were through accidents.[iii] Which, when considering there are over 88,000 separate passenger flights each day, is a staggeringly low percentage. Especially when you consider that there are from 200,000 to 400,000 deaths by medical error annually in the USA alone[iv].

As Zig Ziglar always said, 'Failure is an event, not a person.'

CHAPTER 16

PUSH FORWARD

In 2016 I had an interesting idea.

Why not get some form of training for the barbers themselves? I thought. *That way, they could be more prepared and confident when it comes to certain situations and opportunities to help people.*

I was told about a lot of different training programmes and courses by lots of different people. In fact, I was inundated with emails and offers of help, education, training, courses, and ideas. People wanted to get involved and they wanted to suggest ways in which we could grow. And throughout all of this, there was one incredibly tenacious person who continued to contact, support, and visit me regularly. That person was Gerry Cadogan. She worked for Public Health UK, and suicide prevention was her job. She was so excited by the prospect of what we were trying to do and she felt that she could help me achieve our dream. She played a huge part in getting us on track, helping me to find the right training courses and putting me in touch with the right people.

One of the first things to come up was the suicide intervention training. There was a traditional two-day course, during which facilitators would take you through a process of how to hopefully prevent suicide through listening, finding positives, reassurance, and creating hope. It also armed you with some knowledge on signposting. The idea is that you will be able to diffuse the possibility of a potential suicide by using direct questions, coming up with a plan with the sufferer to keep them safe in the immediate future.

It's a great concept, and yes – it comes with a lot of responsibility.

I decided to take the course, and it was a very heavy couple of days. It was really heavy on the roleplay, which makes my very uncomfortable.

In one situation, the class had to split into pairs and act out a scene in which one person was suicidal and the other would help to prevent that suicide.

Not only did I have to do roleplay, but I had to do it in front of everyone! I absolutely hate anything like that. I just get so anxious and nervous if I'm put on the spot like that. I think this is a form of stage fright, but more than that it's a strong fear of getting something wrong, making a mistake and failing in front of people. Nowadays I get up on stage for a living, speaking about suicide and mental health. I also teach in front of people every day, so I think the difference is having to do with acting in the spur of the moment, even if I'm in a no-pressure situation. Well, it's a lot of bloody pressure to me, because I have cold sweats and a heartbeat to rival that of my fat younger self in the 100-metre sprint on sports day!

I'm sure you know what I mean. Once, I was called out to volunteer in my favourite place ever, Disney World. I was called out to be a knight in an attraction called "Enchanted Tales with Belle". Belle – the female character from *Beauty and the Beast* – was telling a group of young children about her story, when I got picked out to play a "big strong knight". (I pretty much felt at my weakest when they picked me!) I was given a cutout of a knight and told to hold it while standing at the front of the group next to Belle. I had to march on the spot on command while she told the story. I just wanted to curl up and hide.

Maybe I thought people would laugh at me, but that was kind of the point. Maybe I didn't want to fail at being a knight. Either way, I was incredibly uneasy and I'm always uneasy when there's a chance I'll be made to "perform" against my will. Maybe it's because I'm not in control?

One of my biggest fears is getting called out to do something in front of a crowd. I once went to see Derren Brown, the psychological illusionist. I absolutely love him; he is such a talented intellectual guy who has fascinated me for a long time. So when I got tickets to go with my dad I was ecstatic, especially because he had a date in Torquay (where we lived) and I didn't have to go up to London or some other city for the evening. When we got there and sat in our chairs and the lights dimmed, a strong fear rushed through my body. *What if he picks me out?* I panicked. I had just realised that pretty much everything Derren does involves pulling people out of the crowd and having them play a huge part in whatever act he is performing.

That was it. I couldn't relax, and therefore I couldn't fully enjoy the excellent show. From that moment on, I decided that I would only watch Derren Brown from the safety of a TV, iPad, or another device that meant I had no chance of being called out in front of a crowd. Yet for a living I get up on stage and teach and I also do a fair bit of public speaking about mental wellbeing and suicide prevention; work that one out!

I was especially against the roleplay part of this mental health training class, as they specifically said before we did it that 'When it comes to roleplay, do not draw from personal experiences.' Maybe this was because they didn't want us to bring up any bad memories and potentially trigger anything. I can't remember if that was specifically their reason, although I do remember that they had a code for if you had to leave the room, so that they could be there to support you if needed. What an excellent idea.

The problem is that when you're asked to do roleplay, personal experiences are the first thing to come to your head, as that's what you know. And so as the roleplay went on and we were asked to reflect on it, most people said that they were talking about themselves and their own depression or suicide attempts. This worried me a little, as maybe some old emotions were being brought back to the surface. And then those who were talking about their own bad experiences would be left to their own devices after the course.

Of course, I'm not saying that someone would go and take their own life afterwards, but I definitely think it's a good idea to have some screening beforehand to make sure that everyone is stable enough to do suicide roleplay. Maybe some people can be given time out. Or maybe there's another solution.

I myself was struggling to find anything to draw on for inspiration, because thankfully I have never felt suicidal. But while searching for something to talk about I found myself evaluating my life for something to be suicidal about, which I'm not sure is a good thing! I was trying to think of a situation that I could relate to and ended up thinking about my family, work, and the charity, things that I was actually perfectly happy with! I found myself turning and twisting these positive things into something negative. That day made me think about how powerful your mind is and how you can manipulate any situation in your life to look negative if you want that kind of viewpoint. People really do have control over their own thoughts, to make what they will of any situation.

Despite all of this worry about the delicate situation, I felt that I took a lot away from it. It enabled me to feel a lot more confident if the situation arose where I would encounter someone who was suicidal. After the course I was definitely able to notice more signs and I came away with knowledge about what resources are out there – resources that could potentially help those in my barber chair.

It is crazy when you think about how many people might have had conversations that involved subtle little passing comments about someone wanting to end their life. What's crazier is that those comments go unheard, ignored, or brushed over, mostly in fear or panic. On the other hand, this did get me thinking. *What if we could create a form of education bespoke to barbers, to our unique situation? Something that would take advantage of the fact that we often have someone's undivided attention for a period of time, with no distractions?*

Maybe we could create something that was maybe a little less heavy than a full training course. Something – and I hate to use this word, but it's probably the best one I have for this – a little more "sexy" and appealing to the hair industry?

It was shortly after this that I found out how difficult it would be to get barbers to actually attend a suicide prevention or mental health awareness course. With Gerry's help and assistance from Recovery Devon, we were able to fund a Mental Health First Aid course in early 2016. With the course funded for 12 barbers to attend free of charge, I managed to find a location. This was also free of charge thanks to the wonderful Jane Sevenoaks, who I was working with as an ambassador for Exeter College to help motivate and teach their students. Jane managed to arrange it so that we could use the classroom on the 4th and 5th July 2016, which gave us a little time to round up some Lions.

There was so much interest in the course from the media, Mental Health First Aid UK, and all the marketing and media teams at the college. We also had interest from a national TV channel, who came to film a piece about the course. The only people who didn't show much interest were the guys from the original group of Lions.

This actually made my heart sink. It really knocked my confidence down a peg or two and made me doubt what we were trying to do. Just for a little while. I wasn't angry (well, maybe a little). But mostly I was just upset that everyone seemed to be on board when it was all about the media coverage, or when there was little or nothing to actually do, but when it came to taking some time out and travelling to educate themselves, the interest wasn't there. There were *some* guys who were genuinely interested, but being from all over the UK, not many of them could take the time out of work. Some didn't have the available cash to come to Exeter and stay in a hotel overnight. Leaving your shop for two days and giving up that income can make a huge dent on any livelihood, especially if you have family to support.

I asked all the original group of Lions if they could make it. When most of them couldn't, I put the offer out to the barber groups on Facebook. And then, finally, I just put it out there to anyone, anyone who wanted to be part of it.

Thankfully we did manage to fill the spaces. We had a few from my shop attend, along with some local hairstylists and barbers as well as one of the most passionate barbers. Lawrence Fo turned up and brought a couple of barbers with him too. We even had an old friend of mine attend; she wasn't involved in the hair industry at all, but she had passion and interest – and we had one space left.

The course itself was excellent. I really enjoyed it. The facilitators were brilliant and clearly passionate about what they were teaching. The guys who attended were fantastic too; they were clearly excited to learn and really made the two days special. After I'd felt so down about certain people not being bothered, my faith was restored. The experience really opened my eyes to who really wanted to be involved – those on the frontline, the real, everyday barbers and stylists who had experienced mental ill-health either firsthand or through a family member, friend, or workmate. There were loads of them out there who wanted to help, who believed in the cause and in our method.

Once again I walked away inspired, feeling even more confident about dealing with mental health issues. But I was also inspired to create something that was more suitable for our industry, something that was more attractive.

I sat down and thought long and hard about it. I discussed it with family and other barbers and I felt that a brand-new course, created especially for our industry, would suit us better if it was a one-day thing. Maybe it could involve some actual hair cutting so that stylists could learn some new hair techniques as well as suicide prevention techniques. Maybe we could get some of the top named Lions to donate some time and get involved?

Gerry helped me a lot with information, informing me of how these things usually worked and advising me on the normal layout of these kinds of things. I did, however, want this to be look very different from traditional mental health training. Like with all of our literature and logos, I wanted it to be cool, fun, and sexy.

I know, there's that word again, but that's what I wanted.

And so, again with some help from Gerry, I set out to build an effective course. It would take a long time.

CHAPTER 17

SPREADING THE WORD

As a men's mental health charity, we needed to start looking for ways to reach the unreachable.

We came up with simple ideas, such as having Domino's Southwest distribute Lions leaflets on top of their pizza boxes. It seems like a simple idea, but the more people I have spoken to, the more I realise what an impact this kind of thing can have. Sometimes, people who are depressed might retreat into their homes, becoming lonely and shut off from the world. They might not want to go out and might end up ordering takeaway food instead. In any other circumstance this could make people harder to reach, so having our leaflets on top of those boxes reached people that might not have otherwise been reached. In recognising this, I found it particularly important to look for different ways of doing the same thing.

So when The Bluebeards Revenge Premium Men's grooming range manufacturer came to me in 2016 and told me they wanted to partner up, I saw it as a no-brainer.

As things developed, we decided that it would be a great idea to create our own product, a co-operation between them and our charity. It took months and months of developing and testing, but eventually we decided on a hair gel. Hair gel is a common product that many men use, and it's very much a starter product. It's also one of my favourite products to use when styling and pre-styling men's hair.

We had to test a lot of different types of gel and colours in the laboratories in order to get the best-looking hair product possible. Once we had done that, we could push forward with our ideas for design and packaging. We wanted to have a picture of a celebrity or influencer featured inside the box, in order to promote what the Lions are trying to do and help support our cause. The guys at Bluebeards looked into this for us and made contact with a few different sporting celebrities, but nothing seemed to come off. Many of them wanted a lot of money for the use of their image and likeness, so after a few potential deals with celebrities fell through, the guys at Bluebeards suggested that we use an image of me inside the box. I mean, why not? It was my baby. It would save a lot of money and time and would allow us to press forward with what we were trying to do, so we went for it.

We also put together a lot of facts and figures and information about mental wellbeing, mental health, and suicide prevention inside the carton – and inside all of the product boxes across the entire range – so that whenever someone opened a box, we would reach one more person. That way, we would win the fight.

When I first saw the layout of the inside of the box, I couldn't really believe it. I was touched. I had to stand for a minute and let it sink in. Our message would now be going out to everybody who bought this product, and I knew that Bluebeards sell thousands of products, so that's pretty amazing.

There was more one thing we needed to do. One of the ideas behind the Lions is to be able to refer our clients to different organisations that can potentially help them, and so I felt that we needed something inside that box as a signpost. As we had had some contact with the Samaritans before, they were, in my eyes, the key charity to get involved with the product. Luckily the guys at The Bluebeards Revenge actually agreed with me and went ahead and tried to strike up a plan and deal with Samaritans. Thankfully – after some time and discussion – the Samaritans kindly let us use their logo and phone number inside the box. I so grateful to the Samaritans for allowing it and for The Bluebeards Revenge team for working out the deal. It really was a game changer.

As I've said a million times in the past, together we are stronger. We all need to work together more in order to make a difference. If we don't care who gets the credit, we can achieve anything.

We did think about putting a slot in the box, which would allow us to turn it into a donation box for barbershops, but we were uncertain about certain rules with donations. Instead we put the Lions logo and information about the charity on the box, and made an agreement that 50p per product sold would be donated to the Lions Barbers, enabling us to do more and raise more awareness.

I was so happy when I received the box of the products. What an achievement! It was surreal to see all these boxes with the Lions logo on them. I couldn't wait to see how the gel looked and felt. I had always dreamt of having my own product range or working with products since the day I started in the hair industry, but here I was, holding one that was actually going to make a difference to people's lives. It just blew me away.

As I opened the box, I saw my face looking back up at me. That was surreal. Even better was seeing the message inside that we had worked so hard to put together. What a way to reach the unreachable. This could be huge!

I pulled out the tub, ripped off the plastic seal, and unscrewed the lid to reveal the gel. It had that recognisable scent of The Bluebeards Revenge products. I couldn't believe that I was holding in my hand something that we had created together, something that combined my love of the industry and my passion for helping others. It was most definitely a pinch myself moment.

In the first week we managed to sell 700 units. Admittedly, I had to ask them how that was for the launch of a new product, as I had nothing to use as a benchmark. Seven hundred sounded like a lot to me, and I couldn't quite believe that it had been that many already. But when they replied and told me that in our first week, we had sold more hair gels than any of their other styling products had sold in their first launch month, I was stunned!

Whether people had bought our product for the gel, for the message, for the support for The Lions Barber Collective, or for the donation, it didn't really matter. Seven hundred people had seen that message. That means that might have reached someone who really needed it.

Either way, we are tackling the stigma and taboo around surrounding men's mental ill-health, one hairstyle at a time.

CHAPTER 18

SPINNING PLATES

One of the very first pieces of publicity I did was for the *Metro* paper. They wanted an interview and some video content for their website. Of course I said yes, but immediately I started shitting myself and thinking about it any time I was alone, lying in bed, or not busy with something else. It would even pop into my head when I was cutting hair, like a nagging fly in my ear. I was terrified that I would mess up, not be able to verbalise what I wanted to say, or freak out and fail, I suppose. Maybe I would have a panic attack.

But what for? Thinking back, I don't really know what I was afraid of. Maybe I just seriously doubt my own abilities and need a lot of reassurance to get through this kind of thing. I was relieved to say the least when I was told that a friend of mine, Chris Hines, was their local freelance reporter and would be the one coming to film and interview me on their behalf. The date was arranged for him to come into the shop, as they wanted to film me in the environment I worked in, which made perfect sense.

We had to shoot the interview in the daytime when the shop was open, so staff and clients were going to be present. And so my biggest worry was that others would be there watching me. Unfortunately, I really care what people think of me for some reason, and back then I struggled (more so than now) if I thought they were judging my answers or opinions. You know, it was a whole *am I getting it wrong?* kind of thing.

The day came. He set up, sat me in my barber chair, gave me a mic, and pointed the camera at me.

I've just gone back and watched the interview again, and I can see the fear in my eyes. We had only been going two months at the time, and to be honest I was a little out of my depth. I was completely new to the whole thing. I cringe when I look back at anything I've done in the past, but things evolve. It's so important to watch these things back so you can learn from them. With experience things get easier, and soon I became more relaxed in front of the camera. In fact, now it's all pretty normal, but I still worry about what others will think and I want to come across well. Practising makes me worry more, so I procrastinate when I should be rehearsing. That makes me more nervous, because I haven't rehearsed as much as I would have liked. Vicious cycle or what?

I am very lucky that in this modern, technological world, we are able to look back at our previous interviews and reflect. I am much more confident in front of the camera now, and that is due to the experience and knowledge I've gained over the years. Of course I doubt myself from time to time – but come on, that's normal, right? We all do that.

I'm just glad I took that chance and opportunity to get our message out to more people. When the post came out, it was shared more than 2,000 times. That was an incredible, vital part of the journey, and once we'd taken that step, things really started to snowball. From one piece of media coverage came another and another. I didn't have to push the idea at all. The attention found us.

Clearly people could relate to the idea and thought it was worth talking about. I received emails from people asking me how they could get their ideas off the ground like I had done with the Lions.

We even had the likes of barber product companies and brands getting in touch. Lots of people offered help or registered their interest. The publicity meant that we had a good foundation on which to move forward, as well as continuing interest from all over the globe. This alone confirmed that I'd done the right thing in continuing with the Lions, despite what had happened with the lookbook. It *had* been the right choice.

But I admit I found it hard to keep up with everything. I was the only one running everything, answering every message across all platforms while still juggling my full-time job in the salon. I found it hard. I was a director at my salon at the time and, as anyone who has owned a business knows, that's a 24 / 7 kind of deal. I was also having to find time for my young family and new wife.

It most definitely took its toll on my own mental health. At times I felt like my head was going to explode. The pressure to deliver and respond to all the different enquiries really got on top of me. I had a lot of plates spinning all at the same time. I had plenty of offers from people for them to get involved, but I didn't really know what people could do to help, and whenever I tried to offload or delegate some jobs they just didn't get done. I would end up spending more time asking people if they had completed a task than it would take to do it myself. Often it was easier to just take care of it alone.

I still have that pressure to deliver now. We have told everyone publicly so many times that we want to help, that we want to save lives and support those with mental health issues. I realise that this is a big ask, and it drains me not only on the workload side of things, but also in terms of putting myself out there as a place for others to offload.

However, the more suicide statistics I read, the more I felt that The Lions Barber Collective was my purpose. It was needed, and I was meant to do it. It seemed crazy to think that all of this had come from one comment on a Facebook group. I couldn't believe we had come this far in less than a year.

Throughout all of this, Gerry kept me up to date with all the relevant facts and figures, all the details, all the studies, and all the shocking statistics. She also knew the local coroner and a lot of people who had been affected by suicide. She knew everything there was to know when it came to mental wellbeing.

Without her I wouldn't have realised the severity of the problem, not only on a global scale but on a local one too – it turned out that Torbay, Devon had the highest rate of suicide in the area and I'd had no idea. Yet all too soon it would become apparent.

CHAPTER 19

PAUSE FOR THOUGHT: TIME MANAGEMENT

In the past five years, my life has changed an awful lot. I have become a business owner, a husband, a father, an educator, a mentor, and even started a charity. Needless to say, I am quite busy and time is a very precious commodity. I am often asked where I "get the time".

One of the best lessons I have learnt in my 35 years is time management. I am not saying I am a master, and I am sure there is plenty of wasted time which I could manage more efficiently. However, I have achieved more in the last couple of years due to this than anything else.

The first thing I cut down on was the use of social media and television as a distraction: endless scrolling and watching funny videos while racking up hours and hours of box set binges with no real benefit or achievement. Now, I am not saying TV and the internet are a bad thing – in fact, the complete opposite; they are a library of information and knowledge as well as a form of escapism and relaxation, which is incredibly important for your wellbeing. However, if there is a great TEDx Talk with some fantastic information and facts about mental health or business, then I will tend to watch that over some reality TV. Social media is incredibly important to my business and my career, as it is a fantastic way to network within my industry as well as share news and promote our team. Scrolling endlessly is not.

Learning to schedule my life and carrying my Action Day Planner journal with me everywhere allows me to keep track of my time and goals, from attending the gym each weekday before work, to meetings, allocating time to write a book project I am working on, completing admin, managing a business, photoshoots, events, video shoots, travel with work, and even spending time with my family.

Simple things like listening to audiobooks in the car every day while on my way to and from work adds up to around four and a half hours a week of extra education.

We all have 168 hours a week, even the likes of Richard Branson. Even he, with his vast wealth cannot buy any more time! But I'm sure you would agree he has achieved quite a lot with those hours. And so if, for example, you allocate just 30 minutes a day to something – whether that be your career or playing an instrument – by the end of the year you would have spent an extra 182 hours on the subject. Think of that.

CHAPTER 20

SAVING A LIFE

I still remember the first time someone came to us and told us that The Lions Barber Collective had saved his life. As it turned out, it was actually a friend of mine who hung around in the same group that Alex and I did.

I've known Paul for a long time. Our love of music brought us together; we were both into the alternative scene, and that was particularly niche in the small seaside area of Torbay. We didn't have any other choice *but* to know one another really. We were part of a tribe and we've stayed friends ever since.

I have cut Paul's hair for a while now, and I've always admired him. I watched as he set up his own successful business at a young age, doing something he loved: printing clothing. His own clothing brand was featured in catalogues alongside the very brands that inspired him. I was so proud and excited for him; it's always great to see someone local do well on a national scale, and to me he was a huge success. It didn't work out for him in the long run, but he didn't let that stop him! Instead he went on to develop another brand which, in my eyes, was even better than the first. This one gained recognition nationwide as well as internationally, and Paul and his business partners travelled to festivals all across Europe to sell their products.

From the outside, he looked like a hugely successful person who was living the dream. He'd even got himself on the property ladder at a young age (something that we're told time and time again is almost impossible for young people today). What we see isn't always the whole story though.

I remember when Paul first spoke to me about the breakdown of his second clothing brand. There was a lot going on behind the scenes and it was hurting him a great deal. This venture had been his dream and he was willing to do anything to make it work, including putting in all the hours available to drive it forward.

I wasn't prying for information the day he confided in me. I just listened and gave him the freedom to speak. I tried not to judge him or anyone else in the story; I only really heard his side of it and how it had affected him, so I listened with the hope that I could help him offload. I'm not sure if I'm the only one Paul spoke to about this, but I'm glad he felt he could speak to me, even if all I could do was listen and maybe offer my opinion on a few things. We all need to vent sometimes – it allows us to see with clarity once the dust settles.

It was heartbreaking to see all of this bad stuff happen to a guy as gentle, kind, passionate, and hardworking as Paul. But on the surface he appeared strong and, from what I saw, he was getting through the worst of it and "soldiering on" (much as I dislike that phrase).

Paul had a lot more on his plate too. To add to the rollercoaster ride, he told me that his marriage was breaking down and that he and his wife were splitting up. I wasn't aware of this at the time, but he was also in debt, and that burden was really resting on his shoulders, as it would for any of us.

Paul has never been an openly aggressive or angry person – he is gentle and kind – but I could tell that he wasn't in a great place, and for the first time since I'd met him I could hear frustration and anger in his voice.

'You can talk to me whenever you need to,' I told him.

Then one day, I received a message from him. In it he thanked me for the work I had been doing with the Lions.

I also want to thank you for saving my life, the message read. I was shocked.

Paul had taken his car to a cliff and sat there, alone, just wanting it to end. He couldn't see another way out. But then his thoughts had turned to the Lions. He'd thought about what we'd been doing and what we'd been saying, telling people that it's okay to talk to one another and to share our problems, worries, and emotions. That most people are not going to judge you but be willing to listen and help you, especially if you consider them a close friend or, in fact, if you are lucky enough to have a good family. This – and this alone – was enough to enable Paul to go to his parents and tell them that he was suicidal and needed help.

I was stunned. I knew he'd been dealing with a lot and I was honoured that he would share any of it with me – but saving his life was on a whole other level. Deep down I'd always been unsure whether or not the power of my suggestion would influence someone enough to reconsider their suicidal thoughts. Even though it was the whole point of The Lions Barber Collective, I'd still had some doubts as to whether we could actually achieve it. But this proved we could. This was incredible!

Stigma alone can be enough to stop anyone from sharing what is on their mind, sometimes to devastating effects. So the fact that Paul spoke to somebody was huge. It's no easy thing to do, since society has made a taboo out of talking about mental health. Not only that, but it's widely believed that men are supposed to be strong and have that stereotypically British stiff upper lip. But talking saved his life. From there, he managed to see his GP and start his recovery. Now, I'm not saying that everything is fine and will be from now on, but Paul now knows that he has a support group, and that there is something there for him, professionally or not. Sometimes that second option can be all the more productive and helpful.

In 2016, Channel 4 contacted the Lions about filming something for them. By this point we had made some real impact within the community, and Channel 4 wanted to raise awareness of what we were doing. They also wanted to share the story of someone whom we'd helped, which in the media world is often referred to as a "case study". Personally I found the term to be a little insensitive to be honest, but I have since discovered that it's the most commonly used.

Straightaway I got little panicked, as I wondered whether anyone we had helped would be willing to speak on camera about such a sensitive subject on something as huge as *Channel 4 News*. At the same time, I was aware that this kind of openness and the sharing of such things on a grand scale can really help change opinion. Tackling stigma in this way has had a really positive impact on suicide rates and mental wellbeing – especially that of men. I knew I wanted to ask Paul, and I felt that his story would have a huge impact on the viewers.

It took me a few days to pluck up the courage to ask him, even though I had confirmed with the guys at Channel 4 that we would be interested in the piece and I would find a "case study" no problem. And so, with the clock ticking, I bit the bullet and asked Paul if he would be interested in being on camera to help the cause. To my surprise Paul was pretty keen straightaway – there was no need to talk him round like I thought I might have had to do. And so we were all set and ready to go.

The journalist was actually brilliant; they were very kind and supportive throughout the whole process. They wanted to get some shots of the shop, an interview with me, images of Paul in the chair, and then an interview and some clips of Paul doing his own thing as well. It was a pretty standard set-up for a decent-length news piece, and some serious TV time for the Lions and our mission to smash the taboo around mental health.

The video can still be found on YouTube; it's called 'Male depression and suicide: The barbers trying to get men to talk about their mental health'.

'I phoned my mum one morning, and I was just like, "I need help". I went over to hers at lunchtime and just had a massive breakdown,' Paul tells the camera in the piece. 'Her and my dad basically made me phone the doctors and get an emergency appointment, to go over and talk to them about how I was feeling. And it was just horrible. I remember being sat in the waiting room, pulling my hair out and just on-and-off crying uncontrollably. It just feels really lonely at times.

'When I opened up to Tom about how I was feeling, it was more accidental than intentional. It just helped me realise that there was something wrong, that I was viewing things in the wrong way, and that I needed to get help to change that.'[ii]

'We can be that stepping stone to be able to get the person from the chair to go and seek the counselling or the medical advice or anything else that they need,' I say in the video. 'Since we've started there's at least four people that I know of that we've reached out to and helped and saved their lives, and changed their perspective on things. So that's phenomenal.'

'I've been coming to Tom to get my hair cut for quite a few years. I came in to see him one day, and I was feeling the worst I'd ever felt. I don't know if he could pick up on it; I didn't address it with him directly. I just remember leaving there and feeling like, "I'm going to have to talk to somebody about how I'm feeling, or am I going to end up doing something I regret." But I carried on bottling it up for a while. There's a stigma around mental health, I think. I just wanted to be strong.

'I think it's really important work that the Lions are doing, because it's giving people a new way of talking without being judged at all.'

During the build-up, I was a little worried about Paul and how he would react to the filming going public. I knew he was nervous, but I was also aware of the sensitivity of the subject and how incredibly brave he was being by putting it all out there.

123

And after the footage went live multiple times on Channel 4 – and it got picked up by LADBible, resulting in millions of views on Facebook – Paul had actually had people hunt him down on Facebook, message him and tell him that he should have killed himself! I mean, who the hell does that?!

It was a prime example of how evil people can be and how dangerous the internet is. I consider us very lucky that Paul was in a better place and could just shrug it off as a petty troll. It could have been a lot worse, and I fear that people underestimate the power of words online. People feel so disconnected when they write bad words on a keyboard or a smartphone. It's like the recipient is a fictional person because they've never met. But bad words can destroy people – and they do.

If you ever think about slating someone or abusing someone through any form of social media, I beg you to wait 24 hours before clicking send. I hope you will feel different about what you have written afterwards and choose not to send it. We can react too easily and quickly without thinking about what we are saying, and those messages and comments – or even actions, if filmed – stay online forever. They can most certainly come back to haunt us.

Despite all this, I feel lucky that Paul felt he could talk to me about the feedback, and I feel thankful that I was there for him to tell me. This whole situation demonstrated the fact that we'd started to bridge the gap between the community and the organisations which exist to help those in need.

Channel 4 did a wonderful job and I still think that film stands up nearly two years after filming. The piece itself was actually brilliant, and I can see how far we had come in such a short period since the *Metro* piece. I was far more confident on camera and had a lot more knowledge and direction about our goals and mission. We were now making the most of our media opportunities, to let men everywhere know that talking about feelings – and struggling with your mental health – is normal.

It makes me so proud to think that The Lions Barber Collective helped save the life of that wonderful man, a man who has since gone on to become an important part of what we do. He is now a trustee for the charity and helps us with the merchandising. His story has reached thousands – if not millions – of people, and I hope that it has maybe helped at least *someone*.

His bravery is simply phenomenal.

If you are there right now thinking, *I know someone who is, or has been, in a bad place*, drop them a message to let them know you care and are interested in them. It could make all the difference. Hell, I have an alarm on my phone once a week reminding me to text someone. Sometimes I'll text a few people, but it just gives me that nudge. It's not always those who might be suffering. I also text and thank those who have helped me along the way (believe me there's a lot!) and let them know how grateful I am. Who wouldn't appreciate a message like that? I know I would! You might not realise it, but it might just set someone up for the day ahead.

CHAPTER 21

THE LIONS' WALK

As The Lions Barber Collective developed in strategy, the pride grew too. Soon it began to include more and more people who weren't barbers themselves, but who had suffered with mental ill-health or whose lives had been affected by suicide.

One of these men is like a little brother to me. His name is Dean. He is my best friend's little brother and I watched him grow up. One day Dean came to me and told me all about how he had been suffering with depression.

It was a complete shock. Dean was fun loving and always knew how to have a good time. Some of the best times I've had have been with him. I knew of all the troubles he had going on in life, but I had no idea it had made him depressed. How amazing that he had built up the courage to talk to me about it.

When someone shares their story, it can make all the difference to people – especially when it's someone you'd never imagine is suffering. It makes people feel less isolated and alone, but it also breaks down the stigma and makes people realise that anyone can be affected, no matter who you are. Dean told me that he wanted to use the Lions as a mouthpiece, and so he wrote a brilliant piece which we shared via our Facebook page.

The response was overwhelming. Dean received so much support that, to my delight, it motivated him to come up with the idea of a planning a walk. Basically, he thought that it would be nice to get together with like-minded people and take some time out to walk along our beautiful seafront in Torquay, talking about mental health with zero judgement.

What a fabulous idea, I thought, and so we quickly put the plan into motion. Our trustee Sean, who is a social worker, loved the initiative and volunteered to be there for anyone who needed support or information. And so once we got the date sorted – the first Sunday morning in March of 2017 – we put it out on social media and waited to see what would happen.

The day was wet and windy, but nonetheless we had a half-decent turnout. I was taken aback by the bravery of those in attendance. The fact they had managed to come out and meet strangers despite the anxiety issues that had kept them isolated for so long was heart-warming. They knew it would be a safe environment and that the walk could be potentially life-changing. That alone meant the world to me.

The idea of the walk is that we meet up at eleven o'clock on the first Sunday of every month, and we just go for a walk along the coast, come rain or shine. There are no medical professionals there, just those who have suffered and those who bring some empathy and a non-judgemental attitude. We get out and spend some time talking and listening and bonding. We've built up a great support group for a bunch of guys in Torbay, and at one point we even recorded a documentary with Pritchard from the TV series *Dirty Sanchez*, which eventually got shortlisted for an award. Pritchard has continued to support us since.

We never imagined that such a thing would happen when Dean first came up with the concept of the Lions' Walk. It just goes to show that the simplest ideas are the best.

Let's meet up, connect with one another, take in our beautiful surroundings, and forget the modern world.

CHAPTER 22

PAUSE FOR THOUGHT: POWER OF THE MIND

I have heard two similar stories recently; one about elephants and the other about Houdini.

The first story goes like this: one day a man was passing a group of elephants. He noticed that all the fully grown elephants were tied up by a small piece of rope around one leg. A piece of rope which, if they wanted to, they could easily escape with little force. The man recognised that the gentleman nearby was their trainer, and asked, 'Why do these elephants not break free?'

The trainer replied by saying, 'The elephants are tied up with the same size rope when they are young and much smaller. At that age, this rope is more than strong enough to prevent them from escaping. As they grow up, they are conditioned to believe that the same piece of rope is strong enough to contain them, and therefore do not attempt to break free.'

The next story is about Houdini, a famous escapologist and believed to be the world's greatest-ever locksmith. Although I am unaware if this story is fact or legend, there is still a lesson within. He was once invited here to the UK to try to break free from a supposedly breakout-secure prison cell. Now, Houdini had done this many a time, and agreed to the challenge as long as he could wear his street clothes into the cell. Once he was inside the cell, he pulled a lock pick from his waist belt and went to work on the lock. After 30 minutes, his confidence dwindled. An hour passed and still he was no closer. Then, finally, after two hours of trying to break this lock, the great Houdini collapsed against the door in frustration and defeat. To his surprise, the door swung open. The door had never been locked, except inside Houdini's mind.

Both these stories demonstrate the power of the mind. If we believe something enough, it must be true, right?

CHAPTER 23

LOOK AFTER EACH OTHER

Sometimes, I believe that things happen for a reason.

Fridays at the shop are pretty much fully booked, because they're the best slots for people getting ready for the weekend. On this particular Friday morning I came in early to squeeze in a couple more cuts. (This happens more often than not!) Unfortunately, I had a no-show, which is always a disappointment to anyone in the hair industry – time is money, and if nobody turns up, then that time and money is lost.

For this reason, I always try to use that blank slot to do something productive. So I got onto my computer and started to go through my emails, trying to make a dent in my full inbox. This was still pretty early days for the Lions, so I was getting a lot of interest online. To tell you the truth, I was struggling to keep up with it all, so this extra time was actually kind of a blessing in disguise. As it turns out, I then had the next two appointments cancel for that day and rearrange as well, which meant I had gone from having a full Friday to having two and a half hours free.

As I sat down with a green tea, I had a message pop up on Facebook. It was from a young guy whose friend had recommended that he come to me to have his hair cut, as he had suffered with his mental ill-health and had attempted suicide in the past.

He was a lovely guy. I had met him for the first time after-hours; he just came down to the shop and we sat on the sofa and he told me about his life. He seemed pretty successful to me; he was intelligent, articulate, employed, and had had a pretty impressive sporting career at school, even winning a scholarship to an American college for football. Unfortunately, the football didn't work out, and his depression was getting to him. When I asked him about his dreams and life goals, he said two things to me: he wanted a family and a Ford Mustang. I thought (still do, actually) that that was pretty reasonable, even though a Mustang might not be the best family car. After that, this lad continued to come to the shop to have his hair cut. Not only was he a kind, gentle romantic, but we got on well. We would discuss all sorts of things, ranging from the best Disney film to what tattoo he was going to get next. It seemed to always revolve around lions!

The message he sent me that morning took me by surprise, and sent that heat wave of anxiety all over my body.

I don't want to live anymore.

He told me that he was drinking heavily and had taken every pill available in the house. He'd tried to do this before and it had seriously damaged his insides; apparently the doctors had told him that he had a very resilient liver and stomach. It had pretty much saved his life in the past.

This worried me. Would he take even more pills to combat this?

What do you do in this situation?

Now I think I was lucky that my clients had cancelled. It meant that I happened to be online at the right time for him. I can't begin to imagine how I would have felt if I had found the message at eight o'clock that night when I finished work.

I've been in a situation before where I've received a text from an unknown number in the middle of the night while I was sleeping. The message read, *I have been meaning to contact you for a while, but the voices are telling me I need to speak to you now!* When I woke for the gym at five o'clock, my heart sank straightaway. I was choked and panicky, and then the adrenaline kicked in and I tried frantically to call and text this mystery person back. I continued to message them with relevant information and signposting to services, but got no reply. I will never know who that was; I will never know if they are still suffering or if they are even alive. Was it someone I knew, or someone from the other side of the country? If so, how did they get my number? It is a pretty helpless place to be, for both involved. They felt like they could open up to me but I wasn't there at their time of need. I'll never forget that. I just hope they're okay.

In this situation, I was lucky enough to be available. But what could I do?

I tried to reassure him and try to find out what had brought this on, at the same time trying to get him to agree to a plan to save his life. This wasn't easy; he kept asking me not to call the police or an ambulance, even though I wasn't sure of his address. I didn't want to lose his trust by doing what he had asked me not to do, but more importantly I didn't want to lose him.

I'm feeling sleepy, he wrote. *I'm going to take a lie down.*

It was seriously scary. I tried to keep him talking so that he'd stay awake.

Then the shop phone rang. Thankfully it was the friend who had referred him to me in the first place. He was also talking to our overdosing friend and he knew his address.

We discussed what we should do, and we decided that he would call an ambulance and just get them there ASAP. The guy hadn't asked his friend not to, and therefore we weren't betraying his trust.

It is such an awful situation to be in as, like the Samaritans, I believe that people have the right to die if that is their choice. But I also feel that it is important to try to save a life where possible, especially because all the suicide-attempt survivors – or professionals who have spoken to survivors themselves – have told me that they regretted the decision to end their life once they had gone through with the attempt.

As we waited for the ambulance to arrive, I kept in touch with my overdosing friend and our mutual connection. I had to keep leaving the computer for brief stints because of phone calls to the shop and other business-y things that I couldn't avoid. During that time the ambulance turned up, and when I came back to the chat after three minutes or so, I discovered that he had refused help and had sent them away. Paramedics are unable to help the person in need without consent, especially if they're on their own property.

With this news coming from his friend on one chat, he told me on the other, *I think I might go out for a walk. Someone just sent an ambulance here and I don't want anyone to find me.* Maybe he realised that we were trying to save his life and he was determined to end it.

SHIT, SHIT, SHIT!

What the hell were we going to do if we couldn't find him?

I knew that Gerry might have a good idea of what to do and where to go from here, so I gave her a call. Gerry knew of the guy in question (of course she did – she was like the guru of mental wellbeing in the borough of Torbay!) and she said, 'Look – it might be a good thing that he's left the house. If we call the police and let them know, they will be able to help him because he is out in public and he doesn't have to know that we've called them.'

That was it – I was on the phone straightaway with a description and all the info I could possibly give them. The police were brilliant, jumping straight into action to try to prevent his death.

I felt a big sense of relief. I finally felt that I'd put something into action to save my friend's life.

From this point on it's all a bit of a blur. Within seconds of the call finishing, I checked my messenger to see that he had said his goodbyes to me, just as my next client walked through the door. That was it.

I was busy all day long – and when I say busy, I mean I had non-stop clients all day, with no break for food and barely a glass of water. For those who don't know, in the hair industry we tend to book our days out back-to-back. If you're lucky enough to have an assistant or two in the shop, they might wash the client's hair while you grab something to eat, but you're generally one-to-one with your clients all day, since they are purchasing your skills and your time. That means that there really isn't any time to check phones or messages.

My mind was racing all day. *Did they find him? Is he okay? Should I have called the police? Should I have cancelled my clients and gone to find him myself? Is he in hospital?* I had no idea what was going on, but all day long I had to put up a front and cut hair with a smile.

As soon as I put down my hair tools for the day, I was straight onto my phone to check my messages. There was nothing from the guy who had been feeling suicidal. I searched frantically through my inbox, looking for some news. Eventually I found a message from his friend, letting me know that the man had been found, successfully saved from his overdose. He would be spending some time in hospital.

To say I was relieved was an understatement to say the least! Not only was I happy that a life had been saved, but he was my friend because of The Lions Barber Collective. Our whole thing is suicide prevention!

I'm not going to lie, I certainly felt some pressure because of that. How could I go on with the project if I couldn't help prevent someone from suicide?

The longer I worked with The Lions Barber Collective, the more I came to realise that the likelihood of finding myself in this situation and losing someone linked to the charity would only increase.

I now understand that a person's life is their own and they have the right to end it if they wish, no matter how much I believe that suicide is preventable. Samaritans will in fact sit and listen to someone on a call as they die if that person does not want to live anymore, as they state on their website: 'We hope that, through talking to us, you'll get to a place where you see your situation in a different light. But we respect your freedom to make your own decisions, including the decision to take your own life. We'll continue to talk with you if you've taken action to end your life.'[vi]

Now, that must be so difficult. But it must be comforting to know that you helped that person through their last moments. However, I personally hope that we can help people see that their problems or worries are only temporary. Suicide is a permanent "solution", but it doesn't have to be the only option.

After a few days had passed, during which we had a lot of conversations online, my friend was back in my chair. It was so good to see him, and I was relieved that he had a more positive outlook.

'Do you think you would ever attempt it again?' I asked him frankly.

'I feel okay now,' he said quietly. 'But I can't say that I wouldn't try in the future, if it gets that bad again. Sometimes I just think everyone would be better off without me.'

Feeling shocked, I was nevertheless grateful that he felt safe enough to tell me this. I knew that he appreciated my help and would appreciate it in the future.

That really opened my eyes to the nature of recovery. Even if you survive a suicide attempt once and feel better afterwards, the fact is that depression comes and goes. It can drag you down into the deepest of depths even after you feel recovered. That is why I think it's so bloody important that we look after each other.

CHAPTER 24

POINTS OF LIGHT

One day in early 2017, I received one of those phone calls that comes completely out of the blue.

There I was, cutting hair just like on any other day. And just like any other day, a member of the team answered and brought the phone over to me. 'There's someone on the phone for you,' he said.

'Who is it?' I asked, as ever. 'Can you take a message for me?'

'Well, not really,' my colleague replied. 'You might want to take this. It's 10 Downing Street!'

My client and I stared at each other through the mirror, utterly shocked. He motioned for me to take the call, and so shaking slightly from a rush of blood to the head, I did.

As it turned out, the Prime Minister's office had heard about The Lions Barber Collective and were incredibly impressed with what we had achieved. They wanted a phone interview with me to create a case study, and to see if I would be eligible for any awards, recognition, or potential support from them. Of course I agreed, and scheduled a 45-minute call for later on in the week.

I felt nervous and anxious in the run-up to the call, so I kept myself busy. It went on for over an hour as the government representative and I discussed all that our team had done and our future plans for the Lions.

We finished the interview with another 10 minutes or so of talking about personal experiences, and I really enjoyed the call. They went away to develop the case study ready for review, and after a while I got so busy behind the chair and with the charity that I almost forgot about the whole thing. In all honesty, I felt that nothing would come of the case study.

But then I received another call, and my heart almost stopped. Well, it definitely jumped up into my throat! Downing Street had some good news for me: they wanted to give me a Points of Light award for outstanding voluntary work!

On top of this, the Prime Minister Theresa May had given the Lions her personal endorsement. Now, it doesn't matter here what anyone's opinion of her and Parliament might be. We had just received recognition from the highest office in the land. Bugger me!

The lady on the phone continued to speak, but I didn't really hear any of it after that point. All I could think about was how proud my Grandad Billy would have been if he was still here.

What an achievement! It was all so surreal.

The day I received a letter and certificate from Theresa May was fantastic. I even received a Christmas card that year too. I mean, I'm probably just on an automatic mailing list now, but jeez, I still got a Christmas card from the PM!

Of course, none of this is about the award, but it was lovely to be recognised for all the hours and work that had been put in, especially when it wasn't an award we'd applied for. It meant an awful lot and put a spring in my step for days. Looking back and reflecting again on the stature of it, I have even more amazement and pride than I did then. Writing this book has given me that ability to reflect on the importance of some of the big moments of the past couple of years. Recognition is always lovely, especially when you've poured your heart and energy into something. In this day and age we're always looking forward and waiting for the next big thing to happen so that we can post it on social media, or buying the next materialistic object that is better than what we currently have. This was true of me in that moment – I was always looking forward to what's next. There were so many other things going on at that point that I moved on very quickly, continuing to juggle my workload. And so this book has helped me reassess what's important in my life and focus on the Lions' progress.

The recognition didn't stop there. In 2018, I noticed that there was an awards ceremony being run by *Modern Barber* magazine. The awards were called MOBAAs (The Modern Barber Awards) and I saw that they had a category for innovation.

In 2017 we had actually made the finals of the Most Wanted Awards by *Creative HEAD* magazine for innovation, but we'd lost out at the finals. Although this was a little upsetting – I don't think I really believed I would pick up the award at such a huge ceremony, with such big competition – just being recognised was huge enough deal for me and the Lions.

There was something particularly special about getting recognition from my own industry, from the people who I felt could actually really help those in the chair – and men all around the world.

I knew we might not win, but I did feel that we deserved to, for all the hard work that we'd put in. We'd taken the time to stick with what we believed in and used the barber chair as a place to help others. *To hell with it*, I thought, putting my entry together and sending it off to *Modern Barber*. As is characteristic of me, I forgot about it for a while as I had a busy couple of months. Time flew by, and so I was shocked when they announced that The Lions Barber Collective had been announced as a finalist!

I first saw it on Instagram; *Modern Barber* magazine had put all the finalists up on their page for each category and someone sent me the post as a message. I had to check my notifications and check their page before I could believe that it was real. I had a real moment of shock. We now had a chance to win an industry award, to be recognised by a fantastic magazine and a real pillar of our industry. I still had doubt that we'd win it, but I still felt a rush of excitement.

In fact, I was over the moon, but we were up against some stiff competition. In particular there was Armour to Barber, a new organisation run by a wonderful man called Liam Hamilton, who had helped the Lions out a lot. His venture was to help ex-military personnel find a new career in barbering through donations of barbering tools and opportunities.

At last the week of the big day came, and I headed up to London with Graham Miles and Ashley Hamilton, both of whom are my good friends and trustees for the charity. I always like a road trip with my friends, especially when it's a clear, sunny day. We drove along the A303, taking in the scenery and the beautiful countryside. I always find it's a real good bonding opportunity between friends, to spend some time discussing new ideas for the charity. We always seem to come up with something when travelling together. There is something especially nice about being in a car with just your friends and with no interruptions or outside interference. It's just you guys together.

We stayed in Westminster, but that night some of the guys from Pall Mall Barbers and the Lions were about, so we went and met them. We had a late night that night, as we spent some good time catching up and discussing mental health and everyone's thoughts on it. Everyone discussed their own issues and problems, most of which everyone could relate to. Some of their issues were job related, some were relationship related, and others just had daily personal struggles. One of the guys there was feeling the pressure of starting a family with his partner, and he asked for my input on having children.

It was nice to see everyone bond and open up so freely and easily, simply because they knew it was a safe environment.

It wasn't quite like a support group session, and we laughed and joked and talked about lots of other things, but when something came up we openly discussed it.

It seems that every time I go anywhere at all, I end up talking about suicide and mental health. I admit that for a while I found it quite tiring and draining, often feeling like I then needed to offload to others. But now I see myself as very privileged, because I'm helping people realise that it's okay to talk about it. That way, the conversation happens without me having to try to bring it up.

I'm now very grateful, for the fact that we were able to get a group of 10 people sitting around openly talking about mental health means we are moving in the right direction.

The next morning, we headed over to the venue. The event started at one o'clock in the afternoon, and at that point I wasn't really excited or nervous or anything. Waking up in hotels while travelling is normal for me now, so it didn't seem daunting at that time. It's become a kind of standard. The previous night had been rewarding enough for me, even if we didn't win today. I knew that that connection and willingness to share within the group would stay with me.

We had arranged to meet some of the guys on our way over to the venue. As we walked towards the venue in Soho you could see that we were getting closer to the venue, as barbers tend to stand out like a sore thumb. At first there was the odd one or two, and then suddenly the street was full of barbers with fresh, faded haircuts and brand-new attire. There seems to be a few signature looks that barbers take on, including the tattooed look (often there's a barber pole or a cut throat razor somewhere in plain sight) or the bearded look. There's often a lot of short trousers with no socks too.

As barbering is part of the fashion industry, barbers tend to be pretty hot on trend, unafraid to try new looks or hairstyles. If you know them, then you can spot barbers from a long way off.

It is a kind of tribal thing, and it's a tribe I'm lucky and proud to be a part of.

The venue was a fantastic small hotel, with a big chandelier in the entrance and a large, winding staircase down to the live awards area and bar. It was well lit, classy but comfortable, and had a great vibe. We all signed in and received our tokens for our free drink. After the previous night a couple of us had said we would never drink again, and yet here we were this morning, still taking the drinks tokens and planning to use them at the bar!

As we walked down the winding staircase into the dark stage room, there was already a crowd of barbers starting to gather. I began to recognise some of the faces from the industry; there were some huge names there and some friendly faces. I was delighted to see the guys from Hard Grind barbershop there – I consider those guys a part of my barber family. They work so hard to make this industry better and they have helped out with the Lions more than most.

The year before, a man from Hard Grind named Colin Petrie, and Richie Finney of Captain Fawcett's beard care products had organised an event called The Barbers Ride. The idea was that they would get barbers who were also motorcyclists to do a tour of Scotland and England, and at each stop-off point they'd hold a party and a barbering seminar. They wanted to raise money for the event.

'I want the Lions to be one of our charities,' he told me, and I was blown away by their generosity. I'd watched Hard Grind from afar with admiration. 'Do you want to give a seminar at Captain Fawcett's headquarters in Norwich?'

It seemed like it couldn't be much further away from my home in southwest Devon, and yet I was excited to be part of something so fun. I hired a car for the journey as I'd been having problems with my own, and yet still about 20 miles into the journey I got a flat tyre. I had to wait an hour for the AA to arrive, and then I got a lift in a truck to the local tyre place. They were very busy and so I ended up waiting a long time for a new tyre. It was a good job the hair model and I had left in plenty of time, because as soon as we got the new tyre we hit the road and only just made it to the location in time for the demonstration. I'd hoped to get a shower and get changed, but no such luck.

As we'd arrived, the car park was full of amazing Harley Davidsons and a big group of barbers. There were gazebos sporting the logos of all the sponsors, such as Rockstar energy drinks, Captain Fawcett's and Reuzel. The venue itself was on a big industrial estate, but inside you'd think it was a turn-of-the-century gentleman's club, bar and all. Richie had kitted it out to look phenomenal; it had a great atmosphere. After a successful demo we'd had a few drinks and hit the sack before a long drive home, which was thankfully shorter than the nine-and-a-half-hour drive we'd had on the way there.

In a lovely gesture of generosity, Hard Grind went on to donate all the money they had raised to the Lions. It was this gesture that had enabled us to become a charity, and it opened up more doors than we could have ever imagined.

I was eternally grateful for this, and that's why I was so delighted now to see them now at the MOBAAs awards ceremony.

As the hotel room filled out with barbers, everybody started to talk to one another and catch up. I noticed Rachel, the owner of *Modern Barber* magazine, dashing around the room meeting and greeting, making sure everything went right. I know that she had problems – as you always do when organising anything. 'Don't worry,' I told her. 'Nobody else in the room will even notice that there's anything wrong. It's a great event.'

Not long before the awards ceremony kicked off, Mercedes Paginton and Connor Evans arrived. They are two fabulous barbers, both of whom had been nominated for Best Men's Hair Image. They have huge talent, and they had been very supportive of not only everything we'd done as a charity, but also of me as an independent barber. I always enjoyed their company and their work ethic is phenomenal, so I had my fingers crossed for them. Since then they have both represented The Lions Barber Collective onstage at industry events, sharing their passion for the industry and mental wellbeing.

We claimed our corner of the room and we waited, a dozen or so strong, for all the categories to be announced. I noticed that the Lions' category was third in the proceedings, so we didn't have long to wait – and the announcements for the first two categories went very quickly as we all watched on.

Then it was our time. They announced the names of all of the finalists and said a little bit about what we're doing. And it was then that I thought, *Shit! We might actually win. What are we going to say if we win?*

I actually started to panic. What was I going to do?

I tried to stay calm, going through my TEDx Talk in my head and drawing inspiration from that. I wanted to reach people in that room – people who may not have heard of us or would be willing to help and get involved.

It seemed to take a while. A prickly heat of nerves came over me like a rash. I looked around at the Lions and other barbers around me, and they whispered, 'Good luck.'

The representative from Shortcuts, an online booking system that was sponsoring the category, came up onto stage to announce the winner.

'And the winner is ...' I held my breath. '... The Lions Barber Collective!'

Bloody hell, we'd only gone and won it!

Three of us from the trustees board made our way onto the stage and stood in front of everybody as we were presented with the award. It was beautiful and heavy, made of layers of coloured plastic. It was especially beautiful because it was ours. We'd done it! We'd been recognised by our own community, and by one of the industry's finest magazines. I held the award, feeling the heavy weight of it, and scanned the crowd. I couldn't believe it.

It felt like we'd been accepted by the barbering world. It was the dawn of a new age of the Lions – and here we were, marching into Mental Health Awareness week which was starting the next day. It just seemed so perfect.

I really was going to have to say something now!

'I'd like to take this opportunity to thank everybody who has supported The Lions Barber Collective from the start, including Rachel from *Modern Barber*,' I started. 'She and the magazine have always helped us spread the word and raise awareness for mental health and suicide prevention. If it weren't for people like her, we would never be where we are today.'

I also gave them all a little call to action, inviting them to head over to our website and complete the BarberTalk Lite questionnaire, which would provide them with a certificate and a window sticker, stating to their customers that they support mental wellbeing. This way we could add them to our Google map and hopefully grow the pride, enabling more barbers to provide a safe space for more people.

'You don't need to have any specific training to be able to help those in the chair,' I continued. 'All we need to do is listen without judgement, and let people know that we are there for them.'

Once I was up there, I felt like I could have spoken for a long time. I was so excited to see that happy look on the guys' faces as we stepped off the stage.

I spoke to our trustee Graham not long afterwards, and I asked him how I'd come across on stage. In the moment you don't really know exactly what's going on, because it just happens. But he ensured me that my speech was good, and that everyone in the room had stopped to listen to what we had to say. I hoped that

that was the case. If every single event we attend allows us to reach one more person, then we are making a difference. And that's the whole point of everything we do.

To be totally honest, the rest of the day seems like a blur. But I was so happy to see Colin and the boys from Hard Grind Barber Shop win Best Team and Mike Taylor Education Barbershop win Best Education. It was great to see those guys who work so hard achieve recognition and an award.

Once we were all done and had resisted the urge to go out and celebrate, we got back into the car and headed southwest. Ashley fell asleep in the back and I desperately tried to stay awake in the front seat. It had been an emotionally exhausting day.

On the journey home I was bombarded with information on my phone, preparing for the Mental Health Awareness week that lay ahead. What better way could there have been to kickstart such an important week than with an award for innovation?

I looked forward to seeing how this would help us create more reach.

CHAPTER 25

BARBERTALK

As I continued to plan the BarberTalk course, I realised that it was taking much longer than I'd thought. I was spinning a lot of plates, and when you have a family to feed, paid work takes priority. Eventually I managed to get to a point where I had a kind of lesson plan, one that was coherent enough for it to be taught. I even helped the guys at South Devon College create a lesson plan for their students that was based on my template. The idea was that, during the one-day course, there would be a form of roleplay between the two facilitators, acting out scripts which would then be watched, repeated, and then acted out again by the learners. It was a way of showing them what could happen and what the signs of suicidal thoughts or distress were.

It also contained a lot of listening exercises, as I feel that listening is the most important skill we have. Being a good listener alone can make people feel safe and give them the time to air their thoughts and come up with their own solutions. On top of this, I included some information about the resources and organisations that people could signpost their clients to. To help with that I hoped to develop a kind of small, pocket-sized directory that barbers could keep to hand on a day-to-day basis.

The class that I helped develop for South Devon Colleges went on to become a huge success. All of the teachers who were involved in it praised it highly. I named the course BarberTalk, and I even made a 360 VR demo video with the wonderful Nick Peres who works in technological education for the NHS.

With all of this in place, I decided that the training course was almost done, and so I decided that Sean, one of the Lions trustees, and I could deliver it to a trial group of barbers from Pall Mall in London. Then we'd see what happened.

To be completely honest, the stress I put myself under to get BarberTalk out there was just too much. I had mentioned it a fair few times and the media had focused on it; as a result, I felt that I needed to do it now, otherwise I was a fraud. I was pretty tough on myself about it and I had some sleepless nights.

In my heart of hearts, I knew that the course was nowhere near ready. But I thought *sod* it, and organised a date with Pall Mall Barbers legend Dan Davies and the amazing guys at the Hunters Collective (a really cool space for freelance stylists and barbers to rent a chair or the whole space for events education). *If I book a date for this in January 2018, I have to do it*, I thought.

I had the right intentions, and I really wanted to do it, but admittedly I had squeezed it into an already tight schedule, and I needed to have a run through it with some students at a local college before I headed up to London, especially since I'd received some media interest about it. The idea was for Sean and me to facilitate the class and get some feedback from everyone, before finalising it all and rolling it out.

But there was so little opportunity for us both to be free to work on it. The sands of time were running out for us. We both had full-time jobs, and I had a second baby on the way. I also still had all of my teaching and other charity commitments to deal with; it had all piled up on me.

And while worrying about making everything perfect, I also realised that Sean and I were only two people. We both had busy lives and we were in need of financial income, so we wouldn't be able to just take time off to travel and teach this course wherever and whenever we were asked. It would limit us too much; we didn't have the funds and we barely had enough time to practise, let alone deliver a good class.

Effectively, we needed to train people. We needed to train trainers, which seemed daunting considering that we didn't even have the time to train ourselves. It was starting to feel like too much, like a real weight on my shoulders. But again I was feeling that familiar pressure to deliver.

Thankfully Sean recognised this in me and managed to confront me about it. He even convinced me to cancel the pilot course in London, which meant letting all those people down – and that's one thing I hate to do. But Sean made me realise that my health was more important, that they probably wouldn't be bothered at all, maybe the participants would even be happy to have their Sunday back.

I realised at that moment how lucky I am to have people like Sean in my life. It's great to have someone looking out for me, even though I try to put on a brave face. He really had been phenomenal since he'd become part of the pride, and I cannot thank him enough for recognising the internal pressure within me. I needed that. I needed someone to tell me that it was the right thing to do, because I know I would have gone ahead and muddled through it, just so I wouldn't have to let anyone down and not follow through with something I had said I was going to do.

So, I had escaped what I felt was going to be a disaster, thanks to Sean. But it was still nagging at me that we had mentioned BarberTalk time and time again, yet there was still nothing to show for it. It had been a long time coming.

And so I had an idea. 'What if, for now, we create a BarberTalk Lite course? A kind of short programme that can be completed easily, yet still give the barber who completes it the pleasure of joining the pride? We can give them a little knowledge and allow them to raise awareness.'

With Sean's agreement, we took it to the board, who agreed it was a good idea. And so we set out to write 15 questions for potential Lions to answer. That would give us a good pass rate, but would also help people get involved with the movement and help us spread awareness. I didn't want the test to be too difficult to complete, but writing the questions was harder than I thought. As a result, we now feel that we need to go back and re-evaluate the questions, as some people have struggled to answer them (especially as they were quite UK-centric). There is always room for development and improvement.

Saying that, we had still managed to launch BarberTalk Lite. Each organisation who completed the questionnaire received a certificate, a window sticker, some literature and a place on our interactive map, to show potential clients that they were in a safe, non-judgemental place that provided opportunities for men to open up and offload. We managed to massively expand the Lions' reach. We even received some interest from Hawaii!

We had finally got something useful out there, even if we hadn't yet delivered the full BarberTalk training plan. It was making a difference and it was being well received. Personally, I see BarberTalk Lite as a successful venture. It helped me feel that I'd done something good, and now people have a way of "joining the pride". We can give them a little something in return, and even though the barbers are not yet technically trained, they serve as an ear for those in their communities. We can never actually turn barbers into counsellors or psychiatrists, but we can try to build trust and bridge the gap between communities and helpful resources. BarberTalk Lite is a befriending service, one that offers signposting that can be priceless to those in need and their loved ones.

The idea of the full BarberTalk course was still niggling at the back of my mind, though. I was beginning to wonder how we would ever be able to develop this huge monster that it had become. We weren't a training development company, and we didn't have the funds to do it. But I was still desperate to get it done. It needed to pay for itself and the trainers' time.

I remembered that when I did the suicide prevention training, one of the facilitators was a woman called Alison, who had her own charity. She was also a lawyer, so I thought I should ask her about the BarberTalk training. I sent her an email and after couple of long days waiting for a reply (it's funny how time goes slower the more you click refresh on your browser), she got back to me and we had phone call. She was extremely excited about my idea and thought that BarberTalk could be a huge success, which gave me a big lift.

'Even though it's about suicide prevention, the training I deliver isn't a charity. It's a business,' she went on to explain. 'But just because it's a business, that doesn't mean we don't care about suicide prevention, otherwise we wouldn't have created it in the first place. So perhaps you could make BarberTalk a business of its own, an arm of The Lions Barber Collective that is essentially run as a business. You can donate its profits to the charity.'

This really got me thinking. This could enable The Lions to raise more awareness. It could help us create an income that would be able to pay for the trainers and materials that we need. I had been building up so many ideas in my mind about what we needed; maybe this was the direction for us to follow.

I would have control over my dream to educate barbers and potentially save lives. It could help us do more good. I would finally be able to pay myself and others for time away from our jobs, during which we were losing money. I mean, who out there *wouldn't* want the opportunity to do more of something they were so passionate about?

Even though this all makes sense, I still felt a little weird about the idea. I have never taken anything from the charity, and instead

I've donated all of my time and efforts over the years. It's only been recently that we have been able to cover accommodation and travel costs for events, which still feels a little weird, to be honest. But since this point, I have spoken to a few other people that I trust. One works in this area of business, one is a respected corporate individual, and one is a close friend, and I've been reassured by everyone that this would be a wise choice to make. Turning BarberTalk into a business would actually help others to help others, and so on.

And still, the actual development of the course remains a little daunting.

Not long afterwards, I was on a long drive home from a show called Salon Live, during which Paul shared our story on the HJ Men stage as I cut his hair. We'd really touched the audience, and it was an amazing event. Graham, one of The Lions Barber Collective trustees, came up with a great idea. He works for the NHS, and as we drove we discussed the issues I was having, and the worries I had about the training course. It was then that the lightbulb switched on.

'What about an online modular training programme?' Graham suggested. 'Like the ones we use at the NHS?'

That was it! Why the hell hadn't I thought of that before?

This was the answer. Okay, I would still have to build it, create the content and put it all together, but it would eradicate the need for any roleplay, as we could use videos featuring actors. It would eliminate the cost of training the trainers and finding those who wanted to be trained. It would be accessible to those across the globe, whenever they wanted to do it, in or out of work hours. It would be far cooler to do it online where we could control the experience but make it aesthetically pleasing at the same time. That would be far better than begging to borrow old classrooms or church halls. Plus I would also be able to eliminate that feeling that we would be training barbers and then sending them off alone, back to their barbershops with no support.

To top it off, it could be subscription based, meaning the barbers themselves would be able to claim it back against their tax. Essentially, they would get the education for free. And maybe it could even be made into an app.

I would love to include a kind of online support group or community for the barbers involved. If the barbers have clients sitting in their chairs and offloading, who can *the barbers* offload to? Well, this is another problem that we could solve.

Now I just have to work out how we can make this a reality. It's not as simple as it seems, but watch this space ...

CHAPTER 26

LOYALTY AND TRUST

One morning in 2018, I woke up with a sense of fear and my heart pounding. Today was the day of the TEDx Exeter rehearsals, also the due date of the birth of my second son. I had felt nervous about this day and the day after, not because of the imminent birth of our son, but because ever since I'd said yes to accepting their offer of delivering a TED Talk, it had been at the back of my mind, pestering me and nagging at me. I had a lot of other things going on, and while I think to some end that they were good distractions, I also think I could have been a little more confident if I had had more time to practise and revise my script.

The mind is a powerful thing. I tried to visualise myself smashing it out there, full of confidence. I pictured myself using great gestures and having great timing, with the crowd laughing, crying, and clapping, all in support of our message. But then my brain would sabotage the mission, telling me that there's no way I could do that and that I will just freeze, forget my script, panic, and fail miserably.

You can't do this! my brain told me. *But what should I do?*

Should I tell them how scared I am? Should I tell the crowd when I first come out? Should I make light of it all? Should I not tell them anything? Should I have practised more? Should I pretend that my wife is in labour?

As I walked in I mentioned to a woman how nervous I was, but she just disregarded it, really. When I asked her if it would be possible to have cue cards because I was struggling to remember my talk by heart, she simply said, 'No, you mustn't. You'll never forgive yourself if you do. In fact, it looks awful.'

Wow! I thought. *Actually, I'll regret freezing and having no clue what comes next, in front of hundreds of live viewers and thousands on the live stream! I'll regret that more than checking out a cue card!*

But hey, that's what they said …

I was originally going to go alone, but my dad offered to look after Abel so that Tenneille could come with me. The closer the time came, the more nervous I felt. I couldn't even eat anything. That's not like me at all.

As we arrived for my full dress rehearsal, head shot, and briefing, we walked over to the building from the car park. I could feel my hands getting clammy and my heart pounding. We entered the building and were greeted by the TED team with excitement and happy faces. I, on the other hand, was like a deer in headlights. They led us through to the dark auditorium; there were spotlights beaming down onto the famous red spot and the TEDx Exeter sign loomed in the background. To my left were hundreds of seats going so far up and back I couldn't see where they finished.

It was real.

It wasn't long before they took me backstage and explained what they wanted from me, which I kind of took in. I was mic'd up and "ready" to go – except I actually wasn't. My mind was screaming at me to run, but it was far too late for that. I couldn't let these guys down and I knew Tenneille was sitting just on the other side of the four curtains that hid the backstage area from the crowd, yet meant we could see the stage just fine.

That bloody great red spot was waiting for me. One of the team announced me as I waited on the white line backstage, and with a tap on my shoulder from the sound guy, I walked out onto stage to the centre of the red spot. There was a bright spotlight on me, and I had a view of the dark theatre and empty seats. There were only the odd few members of TEDx there, along with some of the organisers.

All I can say is that the rehearsal went shit. I forgot where I was, got things mumbled, and clutched my phone (which had my script on it). If anything, that kind of hindered me. I felt like I was drowning. It was horrible.

I managed to mumble my way through the rehearsal. And at the end Claire, the head honcho, told me it was fine, explaining that they have a lot of speakers who perform like this the day before – hence the rehearsal. She was incredibly kind and gentle, reassuring me that I didn't need to worry about getting the words exactly right. I just needed to tell my story. What a weight off my shoulders that was! I was so panicked about getting it right word for word that I couldn't focus on what I was actually saying. I was trying to visualise the next line before I'd even started the one before. I was reciting without feeling.

Claire introduced me to Rob, a stage and speaking coach who had volunteered his time to help coach this year's talkers. He said he could spend some time with me right away, to try to make things easier. He was a tall, positive gentleman with a kind, warm face, and I felt comfortable with him straightaway. We left the theatre and found a spot with a table and chairs to go through my talk. Rob helped me break it down into five separate stories that I would find easier to remember, helping me to stay on track and keep the flow going.

I broke it down into the following sections:

- Invading personal space, relationship with clients
- The Lions inception and loss of a friend
- Can a barber save a life?
- I believe x 3
- Finale

This worked incredibly well for me, and it calmed me down an awful lot.

Aware of the time, I had to get back to pick up our son Abel. When I got home the sun was shining, and we spent some time together as a family. It was lovely. But once my son was in bed it was time to sit down and really work on these final plans for my talk the next day. It was the one night that we really needed this time to ourselves, and my son, who always goes down straightaway, kept getting out of bed. It lasted for two hours! Typical.

I went through and revised the plans that Rob had helped me with, getting them down to a T on a small piece of paper. It had all the hints on it that I needed for the parts that I found myself getting stuck with. I practised in front of my wife, getting everything pretty much bang on. I couldn't believe it!

It was happening, and I was even starting to have a little confidence in myself ...

I jumped into bed feeling comforted, knowing that I was getting there. I actually don't dream, or at least I don't remember my dreams very often, but that night I had a vivid dream about leading an army into battle, *Lord of the Rings* style. I defeated the evil leader. Now, I'm not completely sure what this meant, but maybe it was because I felt like I had gained some sort of control, like I was defeating my fear? (I'm not a professional dream analyser!)

I woke up feeling good. The sun was shining and I headed to the gym – I always feel better when I start my day with the gym. Today's the day, as they say.

The TEDx guys were amazing and had helped me so much. I hadn't really had time to speak with them much in the build-up to the day – firstly because I had been so incredibly busy, but I also fear that I may have been kind of sabotaging myself, almost giving myself an excuse to do badly. I could have maybe prioritised more and made more time to be with them, to call them or rehearse with them in London (although to be fair, I was completely jetlagged that day and slept for 18 hours in a Gatwick hotel). Still, it's amazing how all these things come to light when it is too late.

Thank God the organisers said we didn't have to be there until the afternoon! Tenneille was a day overdue, and our babysitter only had a short window to look after our son. It gave me a relaxed morning to run over the talk again and spend some time with the family. It was a glorious day and my wife suggested I take a walk down the country lane near our house. At the time we lived on a farm, and the lane is access only, so there was no one about at all. It was just me, the sun, and what sounded like a million different birds all singing their song. There was even a woodpecker on percussion. It was so calming – apart from the odd pheasant flying out of the bush in panic and scaring the shit out of me every 200 yards! If there had been a camera following me, it would have made great viewing.

I recited the talk around three times without any mistakes. I felt tranquil, just looking out into the woods, across a field, or out to sea, with the sun on my neck. I felt good.

I marched back up the lane, got changed, got in the car, and headed over to Exeter with Tenneille. We stopped to get a sandwich and ate it in the car park while listening to the talk, which I had recorded onto my phone. We then headed back to the now familiar theatre.

It was a glorious day in Exeter, and as it turns out it was lunchtime break. As we turned the corner of the car park, we found that the whole outside area was full of people – the TEDx team and all those who were watching us speak. To me it looked as though there were thousands there, like when you disturb an ants' nest and millions of the buggers run out and consume all the space available.

Now, I don't think there actually were thousands of them, but in my head there were a *lot*.

As we entered, I tried to tell the person on reception that I was there as a speaker, but I don't even know what came out of my mouth, because she ended up looking at the list of attendees for our names! I noticed that there were some familiar faces straightaway, and smiling faces were what I needed right then. Luckily, because everyone was out on lunch break, the actual theatre was empty, and that meant that Rob, the coach I spent some time with the day before, was actually free. And so in we went, back into the dark theatre, which seemed even darker today because of the sun outside.

I saw that spotlight shining on the red spot on the carpet, and the fear came back instantly.

Rob, God bless him, was great. I showed him how I had used his idea to break the talk down into separate parts, and how I had put it onto a Post-it note – a safety mechanism to give me that crutch if I needed it. So, with the room empty except for some of the team members, I headed out onto the stage, planted myself in the middle of the red spot, and began. I could feel the jitters again, and my brain just shut down at certain points.

Rob gave me some great pointers. One that stuck with me was the suggestion that, if I forgot what came next, I should just stop, use it as time to think about what is next, and make it look like I'm pausing for dramatic emphasis. What seems like a long time to the speaker feels like nothing at all to the audience. That piece of advice alone made a huge difference. I managed to get through the practice talk with a lot of help from Rob, who encouraged me to plant myself in one place and make a lot of gestures with my hands. I must admit that that felt uncomfortable, but it totally made sense as to why he was encouraging me to do it. I mean, he knows much more than I do!

We kept going, right until everyone started to come back into the theatre. I am very grateful for that time, as I felt it really made a huge difference to the end result.

As we left the stage, I was feeling pretty stressed. *How the hell did I do this talk a load of times this morning and feel good about it? Why did I then stumble when I got onto the stage for extra practice?* It was like that cliché of the devil on one shoulder and the angel on the other. One was telling me that I would smash it and get a great response, while the other was telling me that I should never had said yes to this, that I knew I couldn't do it.

Luckily for me, I had Tenneille to help keep me calm and focused. She suggested I gave the talk to her one-on-one, with the hand gestures that I had just been told to do. I felt silly if I'm honest, waving my arms around and giving my talk to one person in the lobby. There were too many other things to start thinking about and I couldn't seem to get the words right.

After a few attempts, I ended up having a moment. 'I can't do this. I need to try it alone. It was fine when I was walking alone outside this morning.'

With that, I headed outside into the sun and warmth and found a corner. I took several deep breaths, told my negativity to get lost, and gave my talk to a bush.

It worked. I made it through, calm and collected. I felt happy and content with what I had done, so I decided to leave it at that and not practise anymore. I had done it. I had got through it and didn't even use my safety net notes that I had now transferred onto a piece of card. I had just turned to go back inside and tell Tenneille the good news when I noticed she'd actually come outside and was standing behind me.

'How was it?' she asked.

'I think I've smashed it!' I replied, as we made our way back into the building.

I felt a slight feeling of accomplishment, even though I still had an hour to go until I went out there. We waited in the lobby by the door to the theatre. I got myself a green tea, as typically I had developed a cold and cough just days before, and I thought a warm drink might help me out. By the time my drink arrived the last break of the day had started, and that was my cue to get backstage and have my mic fitted. I was to go on straight after the band who opened the last section of the day with a couple of songs.

As I was ushered through the tiny doors into the small, dark backstage area, I noticed that all the walls and everything were painted black. I assume this was to hide everything from the audience, but it kind of reminded me of being in Universal Studios theme park. It was surreal. The awesome backstage team got my mic on, wished me luck, and checked my slides before handing me the clicker. While waiting for the audience to return, the band stood alongside me, ready for their slot in front of the 900 people watching. We joked a bit, mostly to cover our nerves, I think.

While the band was playing, Tobit – who had originally invited me along to do the TEDx Talk – came out and spoke to me. He just checked on me and told me to go and do my thing. I could sense that he was confident that I would succeed and I felt the calmest I had felt about the whole thing; maybe that was because there was no way out now!

Before I knew it, the band had performed their set and were heading back off stage. The crew cleared the stage of all the instruments and cables. And there I was, standing on the line by the curtains as I was introduced. My palms were sweaty, my heart was beating fast, and I had those butterflies again.

Then came the tap on my shoulder.

I walked out, just like I had done a few times before, but this time there were more than 900 people looking back at me. As the applause went on, I looked around to see Rob right in front of me. My beautiful wife was sitting to my left. I stopped. Took a deep breath. And started.

Within the first two lines I had the room laughing. Perfect. This eased me in and made me feel confident that these guys really were on my side. They wanted to hear what I had to say. Not long after that I got a couple of bits mixed up that were in conjunction with my slide. But I kept calm, worked it out in my head, continued, and went around to it again, getting back on track. From that moment I felt good and I really started to relax. I gestured, just as Rob had told me to, although I could have done a lot more.

As I write this, I can see in my mind's eye where I want to be for my next talk. That's a good thing, because during this one all I could visualise was surviving it! Finally I finished and received a big round of applause. I stood there, being conscious not to turn and run off immediately. I did my best to accept the applause, acknowledge it, and leave slowly, as I had been told to do.

At that point I didn't really feel much of a sense of relief, or adrenaline, or even a crash. Instead I just thought, *I must get my wife and go and pick up my son*.

As I left, Tobit thanked me. Giving me a gift and a card, she said, 'We'll see you next year.' I chuckled in response.

Tenneille greeted me with a huge hug, telling me how proud she was and how it had made her cry. But then again, she was pregnant and overdue, and those hormones were working overtime (I'm joking!). Seeing her little face made all that stress worthwhile.

It wasn't until later that night that I actually realised what I had done.

I had written and delivered a TED Talk. Wow! That really was some kind of achievement. I never thought I would ever be able to do something like that, something that terrified me that much. But I got through it, and I think I actually got the point over pretty well, considering.

So – the question is, should I go through with it and do it all again next year?

I thought about whether I should include the script for my talk in this book, as I was worried that people might read it, watch the TEDx Talk online, and compare them to see how much I got wrong and where I messed up. It's weird how your mind works. I mean, who has the time for that!? I am sure that you have far better things to do than read this in order to compare.

However, I do encourage you to go and check the talk out for yourself. Do I look nervous? Do I look like I wanted the earth to open up and eat me? Do I look like I loved it as soon as I got out there? Do I look like I had realised that it was the right choice to say yes to the talk, so I could reach more people with our message? Do I look like I relaxed after the audience laughed for the first time? What do you think, now that you know how I felt about it and how I struggled?

People's perception of you – and yours of others – may not be reality. We live in a world where people are always competing and putting up a front online and in real life. We really don't know what is happening in their heads.

I hope you enjoy reading the script. It might help one person who is reading this right now. Or maybe it will enable you to help another person in a very simple way.

TEDx Talk: Barbers, Preventing Suicide One Haircut at a Time

How would you feel if I came up to you now, where you're sitting, and started touching your hair, face and neck?

Weird, right? Uncomfortable, awkward and unsettling ... I would be invading your personal space and touching intimate places.

But if you come to see me in a barbershop and you sat in my barbers' chair, those boundaries are broken instantly.

It wouldn't feel strange at all ... in fact, lots of people find it relaxing and enjoyable. Well, they wouldn't come back if they didn't.

When I'm at work, the most important person for me is you, the client – the person sitting in my chair. And not just because I want you to be pleased with your haircut, book another appointment before leaving and recommend all your friends and family to us.

It's not that all those things aren't important, but what's most important is the bond, relationship and trust we build over time. The loyalty between barber and client is like no other.

Being a barber holds unique privileges and opportunities. When a client sits in my chair, even if it is for the first time, a huge personal space boundary is broken.

The confidentiality between barber and client is an unspoken bonus. It has been joked since long before I joined this industry that barbers and hairstylists are also therapists or counsellors, whether we like it or not.

People sit in the chair and tell us everything. I have one client that I have known for 16 years, since I started in hair. He told me about his first date with his now wife. I was the first to know he was going to propose to her. I even saw the engagement ring first. I was the first he told about both their kids before the 12-week scan. He even told me top secret baby names … and about the miscarriage his wife unfortunately had.

This level of intimacy between men is rare, with few opportunities to open up and offload. But in our barber chairs, clients will share everything. And we listen.

It is estimated that people working in the hair industry listen for nearly 2,000 hours a year. Maybe we could do something really powerful with that time?

In 2015 I gathered a group of top barbers to create a collection of haircut images in the form of a lookbook. This book would then be sold to raise funds for charity. But which charity would that be?

The group hit me with charity after charity – all very worthy, but nothing I hadn't heard before. I wanted something more original, something that I felt needed the awareness.

Then one barber, Paul Mac of Ireland, said, 'How about suicide prevention?'

That was it!

About 12 months earlier, I had lost a very old friend to suicide. I had seen him just days before, and suspected nothing. He jumped to his death.

I never really knew there was anything wrong. And those moments I had shared with him in small talk, that last time on a street corner, I didn't know what was really going on ...

... that that would be the last time I would see him.

Even if I had the knowledge or intuition to notice something was wrong, would I have asked him? Would I have avoided any direct questions for fear of the answers?

What would have happened if I'd asked him, 'Are you suicidal? Do you have a plan?' and he had replied, 'Yes!'? Then what would I have done?

Could I have coped? Would I have known what to do?

It made me think: if I have gone through this and lost a friend to suicide, and yet I knew of no suicide or mental health charities, there must be lots of people out there like me.

I said at the wake to a group of our friends, 'We must do something. Something has to change.'

Never did I imagine that it would grow into this.

On September 10th, World Suicide Prevention Day 2015, The Lions Barber Collective was officially announced to the world.

And from that moment, a fire was lit under me, one that has driven me on to lead to The Lions Barber Collective. It is growing and evolving more than I could have hoped, from a one-off lookbook to a movement that has gained support and interest from barbers all over the globe, from Hawaii to Norway and beyond, all wanting to become part of the pride.

And we won't be giving up.

Suicide is the biggest killer of young people in the UK, with three out of four of them being men. Around the world, one person dies by suicide every 40 seconds. That's 15 people during the time I'm here on stage today ...

Our two goals are:

To raise awareness about suicide prevention and mental wellbeing – we speak at industry events and remind barbers how privileged we are and what an impact we can have with our clients.

And to educate barbers with BarberTalk and BarberTalk Lite giving them awareness and knowledge. We want to arm them with the ability to recognise the signs, then talk to their clients and ask direct questions.

Most importantly:

- *Listen with empathy and without judgement*
- *and then signpost them to the existing resources available*

It is not about making barbers into counsellors, it is more about befriending our clients, looking out for them and being a good listener.

Offloading our problems can do wonders for our mental health, and because of our pride growing in numbers, we now have a wonderful support group within the industry for us barbers too.

But can a barber really save a life?

One day a long-time friend of mine, Paul, sat in my chair and told me how he felt, how down he was and how he was struggling. I listened.

He told me that I put a positive spin on things. But mostly I listened.

It was pretty early on into The Lions Barber Collective and I was unaware of how bad he was really feeling. In my eyes I had always seen him as successful and a phenomenally driven character.

It was much worse than I thought.

I spoke to him about the Lions and what we were doing and how we encouraged people to tell others how they were feeling to try to avoid suicide. Paul went out by himself and was ready to take his life, ready to end it all.

But he didn't. He is still with us today.

He told me that when he felt suicide was the only option, he thought about what we were doing and it encouraged him to drive back to his parents and tell them everything. That started his road to recovery. That is why he is still with us.

He has said this publicly before, and will tell you again, that if it wasn't for The Lions Barber Collective, he wouldn't be here today. I would have lost another friend.

I believed when we started this that if we could save one life, it would be worth it. Since then we have saved more, and we hope we can continue to do so with the help of barbers all round the world.

Now, I believe we need to stop worrying about labelling mental health conditions and start worrying about the human condition.

We all need to love and to be loved, and we all have the need to belong.

I believe that everyone in this room has had that feeling of needing to escape, like they cannot go on. Not necessarily suicide, but that it is all too much and they want to hide from it all.

It is in all of us.

Mental ill-health affects us all. If you have ever felt lonely, if you have ever looked in the mirror and not liked what is looking back, been rejected or been let down – your mental health has been affected.

There are very few opportunities where we are able to spend time with one another, free of interruptions. Let's look after one another and provide as many opportunities as possible to do so. Whoever you are and wherever you are, there is always something you can do which requires no training or special skills.

The biggest and most effective thing I have done personally – and that has helped the most people is letting people know that it is okay to talk. And you will not tell them that you "know how they feel", but you will listen to them explain how they feel, without judgement.

We all have a place we can make safe for those we love and those we meet. It can be anywhere.

This is mine.

CHAPTER 27

I DON'T WANT TO KILL MYSELF ANYMORE

Now, being a barber, you tend to get to know people and their families pretty well. Some clients come and go, that is true. Some use you for that one-time offer you may have at your shop. Others, on the other hand, will be loyal to you. They'll follow you across town – or even to a different town completely – because of the level of trust they put in your hands and skill to make them look and feel great.

This young lad was one of those clients.

There are few clients where you remember their very first visit, but this one was memorable. He came through the doors with his mum. He was about eight or nine at the time, and a bit of a handful, to be honest! He had the mouth of a sailor but sat well in the chair, and I really connected with him. He was ecstatic with his new style, and has continued to come back to have his hair cut by me every single time for the last 10 years.

Over those years, I've got to know him and his mother pretty well. He had an older sister too, and like any older sister he found her incredibly annoying and unbearable. He liked to play computer games, and had a real passion and knowledge for it; he even built his own computer eventually when he moved on to

PC gaming from consoles. He also had a love for music, especially when he was younger, and I would often let him choose the music in the shop when he was in. He loved The Prodigy. He loved everything that he liked and he knew everything there was to know about it. He was intelligent, yet he had no confidence. He would never say a word when he came into the salon; he'd just sit with his head down, staring at his feet (sometimes with a hood up) until I brought him over to my chair.

Recently I found out that he's on the autistic spectrum. I hadn't realised at the time, but looking back I suppose it made sense really. His mother praised the way I had been with him over the years, but really all I'd done was treat him like anyone else and given him the same time and attention – which was probably the reason why he liked having his hair cut with us.

As the years went by, he was taken out of "normal" school and put into a "special" school that dealt with "troubled" children like himself. He would tell me stories of teachers restraining other children and how all the other kids in his class were a "pain in the arse" and stopped everyone who wanted to work from achieving anything at all. He was then taken out of school altogether, which I feel probably isolated him more than anything.

I once said to him that he was welcome to message me on Facebook about anything if he wanted to, and he said, 'I don't have Facebook – there's no point; I don't have any friends.' And in this day and age where every teenager has about four billion "friends" and never bloody gets off the thing, the fact that this young lad could feel so alone kind of broke my heart.

Recently, he was sitting in my chair and speaking ill of someone he knew in class. He told me that he made his life hell and said awful things to him. Other people on his college course treated him badly too. This guy in my client's class made his life hell with his spiteful words, telling him that no one would do anything if he spoke out about it.

One day, in a joking tone, he said, 'I want to kill myself.'

That's something that a lot of people say on a daily basis – I've personally heard it a few times myself – and we ignore it because we fear someone replying, 'Yes, it really is that bad', or 'Yes, I am depressed', or even 'Yes, I do want to kill myself.' But with the training I had received and my work with The Lions Barber Collective, I just couldn't let this one slip by unnoticed. And even though we've made the question an integral part of our training programme – and I have asked it of many people now – there was still a lump in my throat. A firy wave of panic burnt through my body as I said, 'Do you mean that? Do you really want to kill yourself?'

That was it. That cry for help, those words spoken by people every day, had given me that chance to ask him about it. When I looked up from his hair, he was in tears. It was a powerful moment that took my breath away.

I could feel the relief radiating from him when he realised that he was seriously able to tell someone about his problems, and that they had actually listened to what he was trying to say. In the chair, he confirmed that he had thought about taking his life but hadn't yet planned how he would do so. His own mother didn't even know he was feeling this way.

That weekend was The Lions Walk, a meeting on the first Sunday of every month in Torquay when a group of people get together and just walk, for the sake of walking, along our beautiful coastline. I suggested that he should join us on the walk. We exchanged numbers and I kept in touch with him over the next few days.

When Sunday came, I was both excited and full of nerves. I was worried because I just wanted to help him, and it is a lot of pressure to think that someone's life might literally be in your hands. What if I said the wrong thing? What if he didn't want to talk? What if he didn't turn up? What if? What if? What if?

But I managed to clear my head and welcomed him to the walk. It was a beautiful day, and the sun was shimmering on the water as we passed the palm trees of Torquay, albeit in silence to start with.

Remember, the most important thing we can all do is listen. Don't worry about silences. Don't say, 'I know how you feel'; tell them, 'I don't know how you feel; please explain and I will listen. I want to know and I won't judge you.' More often than not, people will work out their own solution to their problems when they get it out in the open, rather than it rattling around in their head getting worse and worse.

We walked a little way away from everyone else. He spoke and I listened for three or four hours. He told me all about his bully, about his girlfriend, his ideas, his feelings, his aspirations, and he even came up with his own plans for the future. He knew what he wanted to do, and it was mostly those around him who were the problem. Unfortunately, this is so often the case since we tend to be the product of our environment.

He told me that his all his peers did was copy all those people on social media. They believed that having a promiscuous sex life, getting drunk and getting high to become famous like their heroes on reality TV was all they cared about. And yet here he was, being everything that most parents would want their children to be, and yet he was still isolated and alone. He wanted to have a job, be successful, and be with his girlfriend. Right there in front of me, he worked out what he was going to do all by himself, with nothing but a little reassurance and a listening ear.

As we sat on a bench looking out to sea, he told me, 'I don't want to kill myself anymore.'

To hear those words come out of someone's mouth is unreal – there's nothing else like it. I hadn't done anything special except let people know that it's okay to talk to me – and that's something anyone could do! It's something that could potentially save a life.

I still cut his hair regularly, and we speak about things pretty openly when he is in the chair. By no means will he be 100 per cent happy all the time – who the hell is? We all have good days and we all have shit days, and then we all have really shit days – that's just normal. But just being aware that you have someone that will listen can be worth its weight in gold.

CHAPTER 28

THEY DIDN'T TAKE THEIR BOOTS OFF

Writing this chapter feels out of the blue, but I need to do something as I sit here in bed, in 2018, feeling alone even though my wife is sleeping next to me as I type.

Tonight, I had a phone call from my sister. *Should I answer this?* I thought. *I'm not sure I want to know what it's about.* I felt a strong sense of anxiety and worry.

A few days before that, I had returned from a work trip to south Florida. My newly pregnant wife had been in hospital and had come home the day I returned, but the next day we were back again. She had the flu and a blood infection to boot. As she's had a miscarriage just months before she fell pregnant with this baby – and she'd been in hospital due to bleeding – it was a worrying time to say the least. How did we manage to get through all of this? We're such a good team. I'm so lucky to have such an amazing woman by my side who looks after me and supports me through all my crazy projects. She's so strong, but she allows me to be there for her too.

As the phone rang, Tenneille and I were sitting on the sofa together, relaxing, watching some TV as our son was snuggled up in bed. We were feeling nice and rested; the flu had been going round and Dad had been ill. It had hit him pretty hard, and he'd spent most of the week in bed. He must have been ill – keeping him from work is almost impossible! Dad is rarely unwell; he's a very driven man. I think that's the reason why I am the way I am.

We'd urged him to see a doctor, especially after what had been going on with Tenneille. But there was no joy on that front. So many men are guilty of this. But he was much better now; he'd been eating again, driving and shopping, and staying up late watching box sets with Mum. He'd made a full recovery.

Today, however, things were very different.

'Tom!' my sister said down the phone. 'Mum's called. It's Dad. We're going round there, do you want us to pick you up? She's called an ambulance and said he's had a funny turn. He's confused and can't speak properly!'

Shit! I thought. *"Funny turn" does not sound good.* I wanted to stay positive and hoped that this was due to the fever he'd had, but all I could think was, *Shit! He's had a stroke. I wish he'd called the bloody doctors!*

'I'll be down in a minute, just gotta get dressed!' I replied, giving off a calm exterior and trying to be a calming influence.

At times like this you have such contradictory thoughts running through your head. There is a constant battle between positive and negative thoughts, between the best- and worst-case scenarios. I just had to get down there and see my parents as quickly as I could. I got dressed in whatever was closest to hand, leaving my little boy asleep, ignorant to the whole event. Oh, how lovely it must be to be a small child, protected by those around you from all the evils and negatives of the world.

When I walked through the door at my parents' house, I could see the panic in my mum's eyes. She was short of breath, and it made my heart sink. My parents have been a team for as long as I can remember; I can't even begin to imagine one of them being without the other.

But I could tell that Mum was wondering if that was now a possibility.

All I could think was, *Why didn't he see someone sooner? Why did it get to this?*

Was it all due to male pride? Maybe he felt he had to be strong and get through it quietly by himself. Maybe he just shrugged it off and believed he'd get through it with a bit of rest. Did he think the doctors wouldn't do anything other than tell him to take painkillers and plenty of fluid? To be fair, that's often sometimes all they say, but I didn't know. Dad has always been a strong, inspirational man, at the heart of the family. It was horrendous seeing him there, sitting on the sofa feeling delirious and confused. I don't think I've ever seen him so quiet.

My heart sank once more as Mum told me what had happened. He hadn't been able to stay awake all day as he was so tired, but he'd had such restless sleep when he'd tried. I did what I could to try to lighten the mood and reassure everyone, but at the back of my mind all I could think was, *Get the ambulance here now!*

Maybe I also felt the need to be strong, to make the atmosphere a little lighter? Why do men always need to be strong? Where does that come from? I suppose we can't all just break down all the time.

When the ambulance arrived, I felt a huge sense of relief. Here was a familiar face. Here was the gentle-hearted, intelligent, kind and bearded Chris. I'd seen him in the hospital only 48 hours ago with Tenneille.

We made a joke out of the situation, you know, as Brits do!

I hope they take their boots off when they come inside, I thought as Chris went back downstairs to get the other paramedic. But I knew they wouldn't. Of course they wouldn't; there were far more important things to do! It's ridiculous, though, it's all I could think about in that moment. I could still smell the brand-new carpet smell, and they came back up the dark, damp stairs, in their huge, muddy boots. But more importantly they were loaded up with machines and tools in order to undertake all sorts of tests.

The paramedics were excellent. They were both calm, well trained and experienced, and put us at ease. They undertook a few memory and co-ordination tests while making jokes. It's funny how humour seems to come out in moments such as these. It was strangely comforting and made things feel more normal. One of the men was a little older than the other, and he must have been doing this for a while. You could tell he knew exactly what to do; he cloaked the room in calmness.

I'm not going to lie, though – I was scared. Really scared. My sister was in tears as the paramedics went off down the wet stairs again, fetching a chair for Dad so they could carry him to the ambulance.

As I watched them leave, I felt a tug on my waist belt. It was my mum.

'I'm so scared,' she said, giving me a big hug. 'I just can't lose him.'

And then, after a couple of seconds of silence, she said, 'They didn't take their boots off.'

I knew she'd noticed, even with everything that was going on! Mum and Dad had worked bloody hard to do up that house; there was no way she wouldn't have noticed. 'My friend had an ambulance come out for her husband recently, and they walked dog poo all through the house,' she told me, with a slight smile. There was a nice bit of British humour once again. It was nice to see my mum back again, even if it was for a brief moment.

This whole thing was a huge reality check. I know everyone is mortal, and that my parents, no matter how much I want them to be, won't be here forever. But in that moment – when my dad was being strapped into a chair and being taken to an ambulance by two men who were struggling to manoeuvre in the darkness, and I had to light up the stairs for them with my iPhone – it really hit me right between the eyes.

My parents have always been extremely hardworking, and they've done absolutely everything they could for all three of us. They have been an inspiration to me, and they've made me who I am today. They have never stopped, never given up. They are courageous and will give anything a go, which has led to lots of adventures along the way. I've always had the conviction that I'd prefer to regret the things I've done than the things I haven't, and that's partly down to them. My parents are kind too; they'd do anything for me and my family. They always put their employees first and did their best by them, influencing my approach as a boss. These are all characteristics that I hope to have, and all I want for my kids too, as they grow up.

Here's a bitter pill to swallow: the strongest, most influential and inspirational people in my life won't be here one day. I'd had nightmares about it as a kid, and I was scared to death of it now.

As my mum got into the ambulance, she gave me a hug. I felt relieved; Dad was heading to the safest place he could be right now, even if we didn't know what awaited us when they arrived. I went back into the house and noticed the carpet – it wasn't too bad after all. There were just a couple of bits of mud. At least Mum wouldn't be too pissed off.

I spent a bit of time with my sister and her other half; we passed a few more jokes back and forth in the only way men know how to act in this kind of situation. I then went back home to my wife and sat in silence for a bit, trying to distract myself with social media.

It'll be fine, I told myself. *Dad's probably just delirious from the fever.*

I spoke to Tenneille about what had happened, and then I thought, *I should text Mum about the carpet*. So I did. I can just imagine her face as she read it.

'I can't go to bed yet, with this on my mind,' I said to Tenneille, but then it seemed like a good idea. And so I got into bed and took a sleeping pill, answering some emails to free up my mind. An hour later, as I went to put my laptop down, I saw that we now had a family WhatsApp group. How had we not had one before?

Through the group I learnt that there was no blood on Dad's brain, but the CT scan showed a white spot. That meant that he could have had a stroke; equally it could have meant that he had moved while in the machine. My heart sank, but then I read a message from Mum.

I can't bear it if I've lost him.

My heart really did hit rock bottom then. If Mum was lost, and Dad was gone, where the hell would I be?

This point of the story takes me up to right here, right now, in this moment. The latest message I've received reads, *He is sleeping now*, but here I am, sitting here with no one to talk to. So I'm talking to you.

I need to speak to someone and offload these thoughts. I also need to get some sleep and rest my mind, but I can't see that happening any time soon.

We all worry about losing loved ones. I used to worry about it all the time as a kid. As I've said before, I'd lie in bed thinking, *I don't want to lose my mum and dad!*, sobbing as I did so. Now the reality of what's happened tonight is even scarier. It's hard not to think the worst, even when I know my mind is just getting carried away.

The biggest thing that grabbed my attention tonight was our constant use of humour to lighten the mood, especially the men. Perhaps this is a symptom of male pride. I've just looked into this a little, and as it turns out, Freud said that humour is a healthy way for our brains to cope with stress. George Vaillant also stated that humour was a very effective coping strategy used by professional men.

And then I found this quote from one of my dad's favourite movie stars. I wouldn't even know who he was if it wasn't for Dad.

"If it weren't for the brief respite we give the world with our foolishness, the world would see mass suicide in numbers that compare favourably with the death rate of lemmings."

(Groucho Marx)

That quote couldn't be more on point, especially in the context of this story and book overall. We do spend an awful lot of time surrounded by negativity, whether it's at the hands of ourselves or others.

It's funny what you come to realise when you reflect on what is happening in the now, rather than looking to the future or the past. If I hadn't had sat here and written this chapter, I wouldn't have found the quote or reviewed what had just happened to my family. I need to take some positives from it.

I've noticed how close and strong our family are. And when we're together, we're good at coping with stress and making jokes to make ourselves feel better. It makes me feel lucky that we have one another, whatever happens.

But we need the bad times to appreciate the good. Bad times are an essential part of life, and we live in a time when the media is constantly putting out this message that we all need to be happy all the time. But what does it even mean to be happy? In this day and age, "happiness" seems to mean *more*. More stuff, more money, more lovers, more friends, more likes. But actually, often we do better with less.

Just think about when you go out for a meal. If you have a menu with 50 choices on it, it's almost impossible to choose. And then when you do, you worry that you haven't made the right choice, wondering whether the person next to you made a better choice than you. But if you go for a taster menu, with maybe just a couple of choices along the way, you'll find the decision-making easier and enjoy the outcome more!

It really is valuable to learn to desire the things you have, rather than making yourself unhappy chasing the things you don't – especially if you're lucky enough to have a great family.

CHAPTER 29

TRULY LISTEN

Recently I've been listening to music that I used to listen to a lot growing up, including bands such as Papa Roach or Linkin Park. They sang openly about mental health and suicide and there was a lot of hurt and pain in their songs. They vented their own problems and aired their issues and suffering for everyone to hear. Fifteen years ago I would just listen to the tune and enjoy it for what it was at face value. I don't think I ever really thought about the lyrics and what they actually meant. I never considered that the performers might actually be suffering. I mean, why would they be? They had everything I wanted at that age – fame, a platform from which to sell their music to millions, and anything money could buy.

But reflecting on these songs today makes me realise that we can talk all we want – putting our misery out there for everyone to read, hear, or even sing along to – but until people truly listen, they will miss so much. Even if they know every lyric off by heart.

Yes, it is important that we provide safe spaces in which people can open up and offload in a non-judgemental manner. But if people are putting it out there and we're not truly listening, then we won't see what's in plain sight.

Linkin Park's lead vocalist Chester Bennington took his own life in 2017. It was a shock for most people, but if you look back at his song lyrics, actually his suffering is plain for everyone to see. Maybe we don't expect someone of that level of success to suffer, but imagine trying to tell someone you are suffering when everyone assumes you have everything. That must be so lonely.

Like I said in my TED Talk, mental ill-health affects us all. That term doesn't just cover diagnosable labels and conditions; it also refers to any thought of struggle or pain. I'm pretty sure most reading this would have spent at least one night lying awake in bed thinking about all sorts of shit. *Did I do okay on that exam? Does she like me? Why didn't he text back? I wish I hadn't said that! Why did they ignore me? Why is life so unfair? I loved them so much! I knew I shouldn't have told them!* I know I've thought all those things myself, and they all affect our mental health in some way.

We all have a mind. We all need to be aware of this, and look after one another.

Human beings are very insular creatures and we find it difficult to understand the world through other people's points of view – after all, we will only ever see it through our own. But if we can slow down and take a step back, reflect on situations before reacting, and try to have empathy and understanding for others, we can make a huge difference.

Truly listen without judgement.

Together we are stronger.

CHAPTER 30

PAUSE FOR THOUGHT: DISNEY

So, there I was, standing in a crowd, turning away from the point of focus and staring into the faces of those who gathered behind me. I saw people singing out loud at the top of their voices with smiles that their faces could barely contain. Grown men with tattoos and beards with a tear in their eyes and their excited son or daughter on their shoulders. Everyone in this one place was united in happiness, by their connection and love for something created by one man's dream. And all this before breakfast!

It is no secret I'm a self-confessed Disney fan. I love the films, the theme parks, their culture and the man himself. I proposed to my wife on the Big Thunder Mountain rollercoaster. I had my stag do in Disneyland Paris, and we honeymooned in Walt Disney World Florida with our first child, who has a Disney reference in his name. Needless to say, Disney has had a huge impact on mine and my family's life.

On my last visit to Florida, all of the magic, escapism, and love that surrounded the location was more apparent than ever. I have visited this place 10 times now, but this was the first time I'd been with a child of my own. Many have said to me,

'Once you see it through their eyes, you will really appreciate it!' They were right.

From bankruptcy to losing his animation team and then creating his first successful character to Universal, Walt Disney's journey resulted in the creation of Mickey Mouse and the creation of a safe, clean place where adults and children could escape the world and have fun together. All of these were things he was told he could never do. People laughed at him and discouraged him from even attempting it.

He was incredible at focusing on his dreams and not the opinions of others around him. I wonder what he could have done with another 10 years if not for his early death. It is amazing to me that one man's dream, passion, hard work, and no-surrender attitude has left such a legacy, more than 50 years after his death, that can affect so many people in a positive way.

CHAPTER 31

A LAST RESORT?

In 2018, I made the decision to move to Norway.

It wasn't part of my plan, but when opportunities arise, I feel I should take them and see what they have to offer. I'm also a strong believer in the notion that you always regret more the things that you have done than the things you never did.

I had sold Tom Chapman Hair Design and I had made a visit to Oslo to provide some education to the excellent and very stylish Fit For Vikings barbershop team. This time I was going for a whole week, free of the salon and all the worries it could cause while I was away. I was also able to take my family; it was amazing to be able to take them on one of my adventures with me.

We stayed in a cute little apartment and really got the feel for Norwegian life. It was family orientated, safe, friendly and clean – plus the skolbröd was to die for! And so, on the way back from a beautiful week full of hair, education, friends and culture, Tenneille said, 'Do you think we could maybe one day buy an apartment there so we can go for breaks?'

'One day, maybe,' I replied.

Little did I know that just months later I would be contacted by Hjörtur Scheving, the owner of Fit For Vikings, inviting me to join his team as the head of his soon-to-open barber academy in Drammen. I would be there to teach, front and develop the curriculum for the academy and help shape the future of his amazing company. It sounded too good to be true.

I love education and I've always wanted to create a system similar to the Toni & Guy way of working. An opportunity in a great place as great as Norway, alongside Hjörtur, was something I felt I couldn't turn down. It felt perfect, and when I told Tenneille, she almost literally jumped for joy.

However, there was one thing that I was worried about – The Lions Barber Collective. I couldn't walk away from that. I had put so much hard work into it, and I felt like I'd be abandoning the trustees and the community that I had helped and been part of for so long.

I also worried about my parents, who I am extremely close with. I didn't want my children to miss out on being around them. What to do?

I told Hjörtur I needed some time to work things out, but I was most definitely interested.

The weirdest thing about telling people that I might go to Norway was their reaction about me possibly moving away, especially to another country. It wasn't that it bothered me at all. I mean, I hate actually moving – you know, the physical act of packing and unpacking, partnered with having to call people up, cancelling bills and changing address. But the idea of moving away to another country didn't really bother me; it just excited me. Maybe that was because I'd moved about a bit as a child.

After a lot of consideration and some conversations with some good friends, I realised that I could take on this great opportunity and *still* be the head of The Lions Barber Collective. In fact, in Norway I would be closer to London and the rest of the world than I would be in Devon, which was convenient for work and travel. It would be quicker and cheaper too! Work that one out!

And so there seemed to be nothing holding me back. I went for it, telling Hjörtur to send over a contract. Then came the really hard part of telling Chris, who had taken on the salon from me. I still worked in the salon whenever I was home, so once again I panicked about telling someone I was leaving, building it up in my head. I vowed to tell Chris before anyone else, on the day I signed my contract.

I stayed awake late into the night before, worrying about upsetting Chris. I was going to do it first thing, when it was just me and him, so I arrived early and waited for him. But he wasn't the next to arrive, so I didn't have the chance to speak to him.

I know, I'll wait until everyone has gone and do it at the end of the day, I thought. And so I did. It was just me and him there as he cashed up. I stood there talking to him, engaging in random chitchat, all the time thinking, *Tell him, then. Tell him now!*

Then there was an awkward silence as I tried to say the words ...

'See ya tomorrow, man!' I called instead.

'Later!' Chris replied.

I walked out and got in my car. Then I spent the drive home thinking, *What a wally! Why the hell didn't I tell him? What's the worst that could've happened? He'd tell me to go early. That's it! Now you've gotta worry about what may happen when you tell him tomorrow, and you have no control over that anyway!*

And so I spent another evening thinking about telling him and a whole other day worrying while working with clients, waiting until we were alone again. Once again we had small talk and stupid chit chat, and once again I turned to leave. As I did, I stopped myself mid-turn and just came out with it.

'I'm leaving for Norway,' I told him, relaying the details about what I'd be doing out there. 'It won't be for three months yet.'

To my astonishment, he told me he wasn't surprised. 'I totally expected you to something like this sooner or later. You've spent more time in other countries around the world recently than you have cutting hair here in Torquay.' That was a fair point!

I felt a huge sense of relief. My fear of things turning sour and losing another work colleague turned good friend was no more. *See, I told you you should have told him earlier. There was nothing to worry about*, my mind now told me – the same mind that had had me worried about all the possibilities of upset and anger. Hindsight is a wonderful thing.

Now that Chris knew, I had to tell my best friend Ash, who had been with me all through the last 18 years. This was going to be hard, even though I knew he'd support me, as always. And yes, he did support me as expected, behaving as a true friend should. Instantly he started planning to come and visit me, booking time off there and then.

'Obviously I'm devastated you're leaving,' Ash said. 'But I support you 100%.'

Telling my parents was so hard, but they totally understood because they had made the same kind of decisions themselves as I was growing up. They were excited about visiting us in Norway, even joking that they might love it out there and want to move over with us. But there was one problem. Mum told me that my nan, her mum, had told her that my sons had given her reason to keep going. Jesus! No pressure there, then. Just when I thought I had got through the worst of it, I was going to have to go and tell my nan that I was taking the boys away from her too.

In true Tom fashion, I put it off for a couple of days and worried about it. Then, on the way home from work one day, I called her to check she was in and made my way over. She must have known something was going on when I turned up by myself, as normally the whole gang is in tow, moving like a whirlwind through her home. In true tradition, the first thing that happened as I stepped over the threshold was the offer of a cup of tea. With a cuppa in hand, I sat on the sofa opposite her in her spotless home and just went for it, trying the rip-the-plaster-off-quickly technique. I could feel the pressure building up inside my skull; I didn't want to let her down. Surely there's not much worse than upsetting your nan.

To my surprise she also took it well, even though I could sense the sadness in her voice. She spoke very highly of Norway and all the opportunities that lay ahead for us as a family, especially the boys. She even told me she'd come and visit, which surprised and delighted me considering getting on a plane is one of her biggest fears. The thought of the whole family being together in our new home filled me with excitement.

Now that I had told basically everyone I considered family, it was time to let the world know with the oh-so-official Facebook post. I recorded a video and posted it with little hesitation. It almost felt like freedom once I'd clicked "post". It was out there for all to see, and the response was mostly supportive. A lot of my clients from the salon were sad that I was leaving and called me some names in jest (I won't repeat them here) but they all seemed to be on my side.

If I'm honest, those last few weeks in the salon were pretty emotional. Not only was I walking away from the salon I had started myself, but I was leaving my clients, some of which I had known for 16 years. If you have a last day at work in a regular office job, for example, you have to say goodbye to everyone on that one day and maybe have a leaving party. But I was saying goodbye to every client, every hour for around six weeks. There were tears, hugs and cards. Three young girls from the same family all drew me a card each with a little message inside. I had done all of their first haircuts and had known them all their lives. They had even bought a copy of my first book for me to sign and leave a message inside. Things like that just prove what an impact barbers can have on an entire family whole family and what a strong relationship you can build with those in your chair.

That last week was particularly difficult for obvious reasons, but on top of that we found out that the apartment we wanted in Norway was available from the 1st June. Obviously it's great that we got it because – believe me – apartments go quickly in Norway, but we had planned to move on the 1st July as a whole family together. Every other apartment we'd enquired about had gone the day they were listed and it was proving very difficult, so when this one came up, we had to take it. And so Tenneille suggested that she could take the boys with her and go and set up our new home ahead of me, as I would be travelling for at least two weeks in June. It made sense and I understood why she wanted to do it, although I would miss them, obviously.

Tenneille pretty much single handedly sorted the house out while I worked away. She took the leap on 1st June, taking her mum with her to help with the four suitcases, double buggy and our two sons, the youngest being just five weeks old. Did I mention that she is Wonder Woman?

My last day at the salon was the 2nd June and I came home to an empty house. There wasn't much furniture; there was just a sofa, a TV, my bed, and a pile of stuff I still had to put into the car for my drive to Drammen, Norway four weeks later. That was a bittersweet moment, like everything in the last couple of months. I was little lonely, but luckily I was incredibly busy, so I had plenty to focus on.

I was excited. We were really doing it! I was happy to leave everything behind and move forward with my family. I was ready for a new adventure.

*

Recently – at the beginning of 2019 – I was sitting on a bed in a penthouse apartment in Manhattan, New York City. The view of uptown was stunning and the Statue of Liberty was just minutes away. Sounds pretty great, right? I was extremely privileged to have the opportunity to be there.

And yet just one month before that, I was living in total uncertainly and I didn't know what I was going to do. I had no day-to-day job and no home, and I was unsure how I would provide for my family. The job I had moved to Norway for had not turned out as expected, and one of the most significant issues was the fact that there was not an English school for our boy (who has struggled with his speech), despite the fact that we'd been told there would be.

I enjoyed the job teaching at the academy in Norway, and living in the city was great. I walked to work every day surrounded by mountains; the fjord was divine and my class were great fun. But things hadn't panned out as expected. Tenneille was feeling extremely isolated with the boys and we weren't getting any time together at all. We had moved to be closer and spend more time together, but it was becoming more of a struggle. Tenneille only had time to go to the shop when the boys were in bed and I would sit in with them. To top it off, we were not better off financially either, despite thinking we would be. The cost of living was extremely high and with only one wage coming in, there was a lot of pressure. Our two-bedroom apartment alone was £1500 a month.

I began to feel very stressed. I would lie in bed most nights, worrying more and more. I discovered the Calm app, which has sleep stories and bedtime meditations, so I would put my headphones in and eventually fall asleep. However, this ended up being a trigger for worry. I would put the meditation on and it would make me start to think about all the things that scared and worried me. On top of that, I would look into my life for more things to worry about.

It began to spiral out of control.

I would worry about money, our living situation, Tenneille's happiness, the boys' happiness, missing my family, organising a life in Norway, and everything in between. I worried about The Lions Barber Collective. Was I too far away?

Then, to top it all off, I had a to make some really hard decisions about work. That put me into an even darker place. I was going to have to make some serious decisions about my future.

When it came to making the final decision, my wife and the boys were back in England spending some time with our families.

I was alone in the apartment with no one around. I knew a few people through teaching and I'd become great friends with a guy called Paul Nicholson whom I worked with. But when I left work I was alone with too many thoughts.

That week I laid in bed each night worrying, fidgeting and rolling around in bed for hours upon hours. The sleep stories didn't work, the meditations didn't work, and even having a few drinks didn't work. I was worried I had let everyone down, that I had put them in this position and I was to blame. I could see everyone having the best time back at home, and that made it worse.

One night that week while I laid in bed, I had the darkest thought I have ever had.

People would be better off without me. I could escape, take my own life and get out.

I don't know where it came from – I had never thought like that before and I haven't since. For a split second I actually had worried myself so much that my mind had suggested death as a way out from everything.

It shocked me. I bolted up in bed, like when you think you've overslept or missed your alarm and think you're late for work, only far more panicked. My heart felt like it was going to beat out of my chest. I knew I didn't want to die; I love my family too much to leave them and I know that they will always support me, no matter what. But it scared me that subconsciously, maybe while my brain was scanning for solutions, this seemed like a viable last resort at the end of a stressed, panicked late-night worry session. It scared me – terrified me – to think that I could possibly feel that way.

The thought of leaving everyone behind was enough for me to make some strides in the right direction. I had been worrying and suffering alone because I didn't want to upset her time with the family, but when Tenneille came back to Norway and things got worse still, I talked to her in an effort to try to solve everything. And so together we made the rash decision move home. We looked at flights and planned to go back to the UK on 19th December.

After I taught the last day at the barber academy and said my goodbyes, I packed our four suitcases and got rid of all the new furniture we bought when we moved there. That was it. Our life consisted of four suitcases, four pieces of hand luggage, the double buggy and the clothes we were wearing. We had got rid of everything to move there, and now we'd got rid of everything again.

The journey actually went really smoothly. We went from train to airport to airport to train, to train and then home, with little worry from the boys. To top it off, the guy on the train got us some free cake when we told him how far we'd come. It made a big difference.

The two hours on the last train were lovely. Tenneille and I chatted and laughed for the first time in months. Maybe it was because of a sense of relief, or maybe it was the peace of having some time together just to ourselves, with no distractions and the boys asleep. I'll never forget that.

We were lucky enough to move into my parents' house and we had a wonderful Christmas; everyone was so happy to have us back. But soon reality struck, and although we really enjoyed living with my parents for a while, they had sold the house and were downsizing, so we would have to work something out pretty fast. The problem was that I was self-employed and starting a new job, so had no employment reference or relevant records. Tenneille was unemployed, I was waiting for some money that I was owed from the previous job, and my new contracts hadn't started. Luckily our Norwegian landlord reference was enough, but we needed to get references from other people I would be working for and my contracts weren't all in place yet. Because of this I needed a loan, and I am forever grateful to the person who helped me with it. I never asked for the loan, but it was given to me the moment I needed it more than ever. You know who you are, and I am sure you are my guardian angel.

If it was left to my pride, I would have gone without a loan and tried to work it out somehow. Silly, huh?!

Time was ticking, and I had a job lined up for 21st January, one that required me to travel. I was also offered more education work in New York and was told that I could visit Disneyland California on the way to the Long Beach hair convention.

I was worried again that we weren't going to get the place before I went away and before my parents had to move. But thankfully, during the week that I had to travel, we were told that we'd got the apartment, with a moving date of 19th January – a month after we'd moved back to the UK.

What a month it had been! We'd been homeless, faced uncertainty about jobs, money and security. But we'd made it through the slump, and things were moving forward again. I had my family back, and Tenneille and the boys had the family around them again too.

I had work in the pipeline. I could see that we wouldn't be penniless. I could look forward to this book coming out (a project that has taken a lot of time and mental and emotional capacity). I had a new dream role with a huge global company, and to top it all off, I heard that Prince William, the Duke of Cambridge wanted to meet me in February 2019 to talk about The Lions Barber Collective. What a huge honour. I couldn't believe it.

Having had the time to reflect on all of this, it's phenomenal to think of the journey I have taken. To have a member of the Royal family request to meet us is incredible. I hope that he can help us spread the message and potentially champion our ideas; maybe it will even help drive more barbers towards the cause and eventually the BarberTalk training. I really think things are on the up for us, and I believe more than ever in our cause.

The Lions Barber Collective can, and will, save more lives.

Being in that dark place and having that thought about ending my own life made me realise more than ever that we need to do more and reach more people. I had had a thought of suicide, even if only for a brief minute. It was there. But things improved and got better, and I drove forward with determination and the need to be there for my family and the charity.

Together we're stronger, and I know that with my pride I can do anything.

CHAPTER 32

REFLECTIONS

It truly is wonderful to look back at all that we have achieved since we started as a little six-seater salon in Plainmoor, Torquay, in deepest darkest Devon. We've saved lives, we've made memories, and helped change the culture around men's mental health.

I do realise that maybe we've over-achieved on what was originally expected of us. But that's okay, because I strongly believe that I should always try to exceed expectations. Maybe that's why I continue to push forward.

I have been contacted many times by people who want to set up their own mental health or suicide prevention charity. People tell me that they have had a great idea and really want to get things off the ground asking me what we did and how we did it.

It's always such a hard query to answer, as I didn't have a plan when I started. I hadn't been developing this idea for months or years prior to setting out with it; I had no marketing plan or anything else. It's incredibly difficult to force an idea. I feel there was an element of "right place at the right time" in all of this, but things also fell into place organically. Let me show you what I mean:

1. It's nothing new that people talk to their hairstylist. Ever since I got my start in the industry, there have been jokes that we're psychiatrists as well as hairdressers. People feel safe in the chair, and there is a level of trust and we are good at listening!

2. There are scary statistics when it comes to male suicide. On top of that, there seems to be a huge stigma around men opening up and having safe places to do that.

3. I am a naturally kind person and have been told on many, many occasions that I am too kind and need to "toughen what I do.

4. Finally, if I hadn't lost a friend – a male friend – I would not have gone with suicide prevention in the first place, and this could have been a completely different story.

Although I don't necessarily believe in fate, I've got to admit that this does feel like things have all happened for a reason. I believe that once you have a sense of purpose in life, you are truly living. The Lions have become a tangible purpose for me, and I'll never give it up.

The Lions have come a very long way in such a short period of time. To think I nearly gave it all up! It's gone from an idea on a Facebook group to a lookbook; from doing local and national media to receiving interest from across the globe. All of it has worked towards raising awareness and fighting the stigma around mental health and suicide.

The fact that people want to talk openly with me about mental health in everyday life is a huge step. It just goes to show that all we have to do is let others know it is safe to talk to us. If we all do this, then we can support one another and eradicate a lot of potential issues. I am very lucky that I have this privilege.

Anyone can strive for more money or fame, but you can never have enough of it. What I have in my hands is a desire to drive forward and a legacy that will stretch far beyond myself – one that will continue to help others in the future.

EPILOGUE

Here I am at 35 years old, a hairstylist, salon owner, husband, father, international educator, session stylist, and founder of a mental health and suicide prevention charity.

Did I think I would be doing this as a child? Certainly not, if I'm honest with myself. I didn't really know what I wanted to do, as I suspect many of us don't. All I knew was that I wanted a house and a family, just like my parents (who are still happily married, though not without their hard times over the years).

I am truly grateful for my life and how it has turned out, and I consider myself to be an unbelievably lucky man. I have everything I could possibly need. I am also incredibly happy that I have learnt to appreciate the things I have already and not take all of this for granted.

Writing this book has made me stop and think about what The Lions Barber Collective has achieved with so many people – including my friend Paul – and I'm not ashamed to say that I've shed a tear or two. I saved a life. *We* saved a life – the life of an amazing person without whom I could not have done so much for the Lions. I am so thankful that he's still here.

I've been so busy with everything I've been doing in the past two years that I've not had enough time to step back and reflect on what actually happened that day. The impact of what we have been doing has finally hit me. I mean, I knew what we were doing, and people have said great things to me about it, but I never truly appreciated its significance until now.

In truth, though, it hasn't all been a success story along the way. Sadly we have lost a young man who worked as a model for me on some photoshoots; he'd also done some work with The Bluebeards Revenge. It was a shocking, sobering moment when I found out that he'd taken his own life. I actually received the message about it on Facebook, from the same person I first spoke to about Alex's death. It all seemed like déjà vu and devastatingly familiar.

I couldn't believe it was happening again. This time it was someone who knew he could speak to me in confidence. He'd received information about what resources there were out there. It really upset me, especially since we'd done a photoshoot not long before that, and he'd seemed so upbeat and confident. He was such a great model; he loved being in front of the camera. Photoshoots can be long and boring, and they can involve a lot of waiting around some days. But this guy lit up the room and entertained the rest of the gang that day.

Although heartbroken that we had lost another young man with so much potential and his whole life ahead of him, I felt even more determined to drive The Lions Barber Collective forward. I wanted to provide even more opportunities for men to open up and offload and I wanted to keep reducing stigma around men's mental ill-health and suicide.

I feel terrible about what happened to him, but I will never give up. Hopefully we can go on to save another life. And then another.

In September 2017 I decided to sell my barbershop to a colleague, in order to spend more time on my family, barber education and – believe it or not – mental health and suicide prevention. I can tell you now that it was one of the best decisions I have ever made. I felt as though it was time to move on, and I had other things to focus on. It meant I could do far more for the charity and for my family.

Since I wrote the chapter about my dad, he came out of hospital and is now on the road to recovery. Seeing Dad hooked up to all those machines in what looked like some kind of alien abduction scene genuinely scared me. It's amazing how quickly the human brain recovers from trauma and levels out to normality once again.

What's truly fantastic is the support we've received from the hospital. The ICU team are unbelievable, and their aftercare regarding his mental health stood out in particular. Dad went back to the hospital to get a full explanation of what had happened to him; things like this can be so mentally traumatic and can result in nightmares. They told him what had happened and followed up with some counselling.

Brilliant. I'm so glad this kind of thing exists, and that it's not all just brushed under the carpet once he's physically fine again. It's great that they recognised a need for counselling and are offering this support. Mum and I are so thankful for the NHS – Mum calls them "totally priceless". I know the NHS isn't perfect, but jeez, it is a lifesaver.

Eighteen months after Abel was born, we started to try for another baby. And with Tenneille's pinpoint timing and organisation, she got pregnant almost straightaway. When the time came for our 12-week scan, we bounced along to it, thoroughly excited and ready with a pocket full of change for our scan photos.

But when they applied the ultrasound wand, there was a long silence. 'I just need to go ahead and get the internal scanner,' she told us. And when she came back, the internal scanner found nothing.

No heartbeat.

I hadn't been worried this time. The first time around there had been a lot of panic and worry. It hadn't felt real until I saw that first scan, that first image wiggling around on the screen; whereas this time I'd been relaxed. We'd planned so much already, just assuming everything would be great like the first pregnancy. And then this.

Nothing. I felt nothing.

I looked to Tenneille, and saw her little broken face in tears. We had been so excited.

The nurse got us up and asked us to sit in the waiting room. Thankfully one of our clients from the salon is a midwife and she was working that day. She is one of the loveliest women you'll ever meet. She came in and somehow made it all seem better than it was. She gave us a lot of answers, but no one could explain why it had happened. We had lost a life and it was more than devastating, especially for my wife.

Very bravely, Tenneille shared her experience with others through social media. It was shocking how many other people who we knew had suffered, and yet we'd been completely unaware of it. Once they'd been shown that it was okay to share, they let it out – and I think that helped Tenneille feel a bit better about everything. She had, in turn, helped others speak about their experiences.

We will never forget it. It was a hard time for both of us. It hit Tenneille hard, and her body had to go through some awful things. I felt useless, and though Tenneille didn't expect me to fix anything, I wanted to. But I just couldn't.

Soon after Tenneille's miscarriage, we were blessed with the birth of our second boy, Drake, in 2018. Once again, my Wonder Woman wife gave birth with no painkillers. We worried about how Abel would react when we bought Drake home, but we bought a big tractor toy as a gift from Drake to Abel, and he was won over straightaway! We couldn't be happier to have our two little boys, who love each other so much.

In October 2018, I was contacted by Psychiatrist of the Year, advisor to the RNLI and consultant to NHS Mental Health, Dr

Peter Aitken. He wanted to meet up with me and discuss what we had been doing with The Lions Barber Collective. Peter seemed impressed with what we had done and how we could use our position as barbers to provide a safe space for men.

This led him onto the barber surgeons. Peter was a member of the Worshipful Company of Barbers, and he thought they might be interested in inviting me along to their headquarters to discuss what we'd been doing.

Now, as far as I was aware, the Worshipful Company of Barbers hadn't had any actual barbers in their company for many, many years, despite the fact that it used to be an organisation made up of both barbers and barber surgeons. Nowadays it's pretty much all medical based. The company is a huge charity that provides charitable donations, resources and a venue for other charities. It's one of the oldest companies of the City of London, and they recently celebrated their 700-year anniversary.

Here is a brief history of The Worshipful Company of Barbers, according to Wikipedia.[vi]

The first mention of the Barbers' Company occurs in 1308, when Richard le Barbour was elected by the Court of Aldermen to keep order amongst his fellows. Barbers originally aided monks, who were at the time the traditional practitioners of medicine and surgery, because Papal decrees prohibited members of religious orders themselves from spilling blood. In addition to haircutting, hairdressing, and shaving, barbers performed surgery: neck manipulation; cleansing of ears and scalp; draining/lancing of boils, fistulae, and cysts with wicks; bloodletting and leeching; fire cupping; enemas; and the extraction of teeth.

Soon surgeons with little expertise in the haircutting and shaving arts of the barbers began to join the Company, but in 1368, the surgeons were allowed to form their own, unincorporated Fellowship or Guild. However, the Barbers' Guild retained the power to oversee surgical practices in London. The Barbers' Guild continued this oversight after it became, by Royal Charter of 1462, a Company.

The Fellowship of Surgeons merged with the Barbers' Company in 1540 by Act of Parliament to form the Company of Barbers and Surgeons. The Act specified that no surgeon could cut hair or shave another, and that no barber could practice surgery; the only common activity was to be the extraction of teeth. The barber pole, featuring red and white spiralling stripes, indicated the two crafts (surgery in red and barbering in white). Barbers received higher pay than surgeons until surgeons were entered into British war ships during naval wars.

However, with the rising professionalism of surgery, in 1745 the surgeons broke away from the barbers to form the Company of Surgeons, which became the Royal College of Surgeons in 1800.

In 1919 the bonds between the Company of Barber Surgeons and the Royal College of Surgeons were re-established and surgeons, including surgeons to the Royal Family and the Royal Household, have been regularly admitted to the Company ever since in memory of the past union.

The Company no longer retains an association with the hairdressing profession. It does however retain its links with surgery, principally acting as a charitable institution to the benefit of medical and surgical causes. In modern times, between one-third and one-half of the Company's liverymen are surgeons, dentists or other medical practitioners.

It was, therefore, a huge honour for me to be the first barber in God knows how long to be invited along and – as Peter suggested – be considered for becoming a new member of their organisation, representing barbering. After a bit of back and forth, a date was scheduled for me to come and meet with the powers that be at the worshipful company of barber surgeons in the City of London.

This would be the Monday after Salon International, the biggest hair show of the year at London ExCeL in October 2018.

The weekend is normally very busy, and I had a stint on stage with the Lions Barber Collective. To give you a size of the event, there are about 40000 attendees over the weekend.

After two extremely busy days, I was up early on the Monday to check on all the guys that would be on stage for the charity later that day. I rushed in with some leaflets and Lions T-shirts for everybody, then headed back out and filmed a brief interview by the docklands for *Russia Today TV*. I then jumped into an Uber, and making my way across London right into the city centre. As we made our way towards the Barber Surgeons hall, I was little nervous. I was meeting with the powers that be; they were all of public-school background and very high up in the education and medical professions. They were all part of an ancient company, one that had held onto the historical traditions for the past 700 years. Would there be too much of a distance between us? Are the modern-day barbering world and the modern-day medical world too far removed from one another? Would they get what I was trying to do? Would Peter be there?

I arrived near the hall and, after a few minutes fighting with Google Maps, I managed to find the place down a dead-end side road, hidden away and surrounded by the banks of London. As I walked into the courtyard area I stopped for a minute and tried to collect myself, and as I did, Peter came out of the hall to greet me with a huge smile on his face and a bounce in his step. It was a relief to see him but also a bit of a shock, as it meant I had to go straight in and everyone right away.

I was met by two older gentlemen and a woman, all of them smartly dressed. On that day the hall was actually being used for blood donation, which is kind of ironic because this is where, 700 years ago, barbers would actually let blood. We exchanged a few jokes about it before we were ushered into a meeting room and seated around a large antique table, where I was formally introduced to everybody and given the history on the barber surgeons.

I was still nervous, but I felt good because Peter was sitting next to me. I knew what a great guy he was and how much he believed in what we were doing. I knew I had his support, and he helped me explain to the group what The Lions did, ensuring that I didn't miss anything out.

After about 45 minutes of talking about each others' organisations, I was taken on a tour around the hall and shown some of the unique things that they have managed to preserve over 700 years. The hall has been on that site since its inception, but the current one is the third building because the first was destroyed by the great fire of London and the second was bombed by the Nazis. They still have one piece of the original stained glass preserved, which was absolutely stunning. In one of the halls they have paintings of Henry VIII creating the Barber Surgeons Company, and they also have artefacts which he gave to them. They had a great display of beautifully designed antique shaving bowls made out of porcelain.

They even have their own mythical creature, the Opinicus, which is part lion!

Later on we had our own private lunch in a room at the back of a small local pub. The door was closed behind us and there were just me and four barber surgeons. It felt a little more relaxed and the conversation flowed better. They tried to find out from me what I needed from them, and I felt that they wanted to have a connection with barbering again, one that they had lost so many years ago.

Now, I'm very passionate about what I do, but I'm not a businessman or negotiator. I felt like I couldn't ask them for anything as *they* had invited me. Instead I just felt the need to show them my passion and how much I believed in the cause. What did we really need? I have always felt that we could raise awareness with very little; we are excellent at doing that. But there is a lot more that I'd like to do – including having a pop-up barbershop to take to events that are populated mostly by men – and I could also do with some help with organising BarberTalk.

As I sat in the back of another Uber on my way home, I received an email from Peter to say that they were pleased with the meeting and saw that they could help us, especially with certain aspects of BarberTalk training. They could also potentially let us use the Barber Surgeons Hall for a Lions dinner event one day. It's fantastic to think that that hall could be home to barbers once again.

It's moments like this when I realise that all the crazy busy and draining work is worth it. It's early days yet, but I'm happy that we might be one step closer to making BarberTalk a reality.

It's been a long journey towards achieving all the milestones I've reached, especially in the six years since I opened my own business. This doesn't mean that I don't strive for more, though – I make new, ever-adapting goals every day. If I wasn't this way inclined, I wouldn't be here writing this book, dreaming of the seemingly unbelievable prospect that something I've written could be on the shelves of a real-life book shop!

However, despite all of the good things I've done with my charity, one of the biggest problems that I'm all too aware of having – and I try to rectify this all the time – is that I spend too much time looking at what's next. I know that that's a big part of this world we live in, a world of credit in which we own something long before we have paid for it. And then we look for the next thing to own before we have even paid that off.

Very recently, I was lying in my garden on my wedding anniversary. The sun was shining, my parents were looking after my son, and my wife had surprised me with a wonderful dinner. I lived in the middle of farmland for three years, with one set of neighbours. There are beautiful views for miles and miles, and yet this was the first time I had really been there by myself, shut off, listening to the birds and the sound of cars in the distance on the country road. I felt the cool breeze and watched the planes overhead, wondering where they were all heading.

Up until recently, my normal days were full to the brim. I would get up at five o'clock so that I could drive to the gym and work out before the family woke up. This meant that I could spend time with them at breakfast and not miss any time with them. I am usually exhausted after work, so I wouldn't make it to the gym then. I would then make it to my salon for eight o'clock(or just afterwards, depending on the traffic – Devon tends to double its population in the summer months, but the roads stay just as small, often with plenty of roadworks), in order to have everything up and running for my first clients at nine o'clock. A full day with clients usually followed, with any breaks or no-show appointments easily filled with emails, media interviews about The Lions Barber Collective, or taking the chance to write my first book, *The Barber Boom*. Occasionally I would stay late for extra clients, but once work was done and the salon was all clean and tidy, I would lock up and drive home (usually listening to audiobooks, as I find that I can fill travelling time with something more useful than the tripe the radio force-feeds you) in time to see the family before my son's bedtime. My wife and I would sing or read him to sleep, then I would partake in a little work on the sofa before taking some time to relax. Then I would get to bed pretty early, aware that I would be up at five o'clock again to sneak out to the gym.

And so, when I was just lying there in my back garden on my anniversary, I realised that it had probably been around 15 or 16 years since I'd last done something like that. I didn't have a care in the world – I just enjoyed what was there around me, without the worries or responsibilities of what I needed or wanted to do. It was truly refreshing and relaxing, and it allowed me to recharge. It was just nice to be myself, even for a few minutes.

Sometimes it is good to take a step back and just enjoy your experiences. It is good to enjoy people, to enjoy sights, sounds, scents – or a combination of them all in one moment.

I'll try to take more time to do that from now on.

It's taken 35 years to get me to this point – 35 years of choices, all of which have led me to write this book. And where am I right now, as I write? I'm sitting on a plane, returning to Stockholm for the second year running, to cut hair on stage at the Swedish Barber Expo. Who'd have thought it?

REFERENCES

i **Samaritans.org** (2017). Crop, look and listen: hairdressers help Samaritans highlight the life-saving power of listening. Retrieved from www.samaritans.org/news/crop-look-and-listen-hairdressers-help-samaritans-highlight-life-saving-power-listening. [Accessed 03.19.17]

ii **American Foundation for Suicide Prevention** (2018). Suicide Statistics. Retrieved from https://afsp.org/about-suicide/suicide-statistics/. [Accessed 15.06.18]

iii **Smith, O.** (2015). 2015 was the safest year in aviation history. Retrieved from www.telegraph.co.uk/travel/news/2015-was-the-safest-year-in-aviation-history/. [Accessed 04.07.17]

iv **Jacob, A.** (2017). Medical Errors: The Third Leading Cause of Death in the United States. Retrieved from www.mdmag.com/conference-coverage/aapa-2017/medical-errors-the-third-leading-cause-of-death-in-the-united-states. [Accessed 04.01.17]

v **Channel 4 news**. (2016). Male depression and suicide: The barbers trying to get men to talk about their mental health. [Online video]. Available at: www.youtube.com/watch?v=68Xq2gh-hQ4 [Accessed 12.12.16]

vi **Worshipful Company of Barbers.** (Last revision date 10 August 2018.) In Wikipedia. Retrieved from https://en.wikipedia.org/wiki/Worshipful_Company_of_Barbers

ACKNOWLEDGEMENTS

I want to thank anyone who has played any part within The Lions Barber Collective, from inception to the time of publishing this book, and anyone who helps us save a life in the future. Thank you to all the barbers who believe in what we do, to those who have officially joined the pride and to those who are a kind ear for the clients in their chairs – even if they have never heard of The Lions Barber Collective. Together we are stronger!

Thank you to my wife, Tenneille, for supporting me in the process of writing this book, the never-ending work of the charity and my regular work. Thank you for being such an amazing wife and mother to our boys.

**If you found this book interesting ...
why not read these next?**

Man Up Man Down

Standing up to Suicide

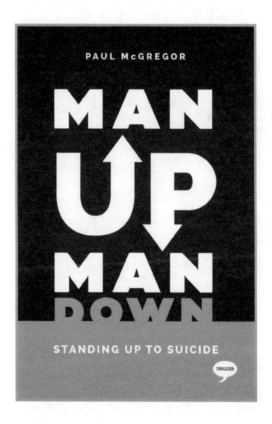

When his dad died suddenly by suicide, Paul was devastated.
Now he's on a mission to change how we think about men's
mental health and what it really means to "man up".

Daddy Blues

Postnatal Depression and Fatherhood

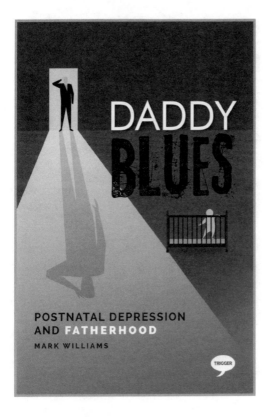

Mark knew of baby blues for mothers, but never thought it might happen to him. And then it did. *Daddy Blues* explores a story we all know, from a different perspective.

This Too Will Pass

Anxiety in a Professional World

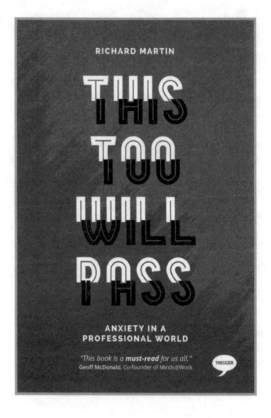

What happens when you have a breakdown?
Can you ever pick up the pieces?
Or do you have to create a whole new life for yourself?
Richard's book answers those questions.

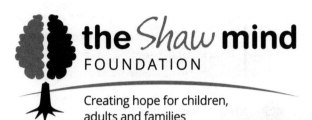

the *Shaw* mind

FOUNDATION

Creating hope for children,
adults and families

Sign up to our charity, The Shaw Mind Foundation

www.shawmindfoundation.org

and keep in touch with us; we would love to hear
from you.

*We aim to bring to an end the suffering and despair caused
by mental health issues. Our goal is to make help and support
available for every single person in society, from all walks of
life. We will never stop offering hope. These are our promises.*

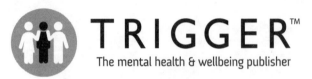

TRIGGER™

The mental health & wellbeing publisher

www.triggerpublishing.com

Trigger is a publishing house devoted to opening conversations about mental health. We tell the stories of people who have suffered from mental illnesses and recovered, so that others may learn from them.

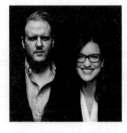

Adam Shaw is a worldwide mental health advocate and philanthropist. Now in recovery from mental health issues, he is committed to helping others suffering from debilitating mental health issues through the global charity he co-founded, The Shaw Mind Foundation. www.shawmindfoundation.org

Lauren Callaghan (CPsychol, PGDipClinPsych, PgCert, MA (hons), LLB (hons), BA), born and educated in New Zealand, is an innovative industry-leading psychologist based in London, United Kingdom. Lauren has worked with children and young people, and their families, in a number of clinical settings providing evidence based treatments for a range of illnesses, including anxiety and obsessional problems. She was a psychologist at the specialist national treatment centres for severe obsessional problems in the UK and is renowned as an expert in the field of mental health, recognised for diagnosing and successfully treating OCD and anxiety related illnesses in particular. In addition to appearing as a treating clinician in the critically acclaimed and BAFTA award-winning documentary *Bedlam*, Lauren is a frequent guest speaker on mental health conditions in the media and at academic conferences. Lauren also acts as a guest lecturer and honorary researcher at the Institute of Psychiatry Kings College, UCL.